Emerging Issues in Family and Individual Resilience

Series Editor

Amanda W. Harrist, Oklahoma State University, Stillwater, USA

Each year the Oklahoma State University's Center for Family Resilience holds a conference where distinguished and rising scholars from diverse disciplines discuss cutting-edge work and foster the community of educators and researchers in the field of family resilience. Presenting research-based knowledge from a range of academic disciplines such as family studies, human development, psychology, sociology, social work, education, law, and medicine, the series facilitates the development of evidence-based resilience practices, programs, and policies for those working with families at risk.

Ginger Welch • Amanda W. Harrist • Haley Hall
Editors

Stress, Resilience, and Healthy Relationships with Food and Family

Springer

Editors
Ginger Welch
Oklahoma State University
Stillwater, OK, USA

Amanda W. Harrist
Oklahoma State University
Stillwater, OK, USA

Haley Hall
Oklahoma State University
Stillwater, OK, USA

ISSN 2366-6072 ISSN 2366-6080 (electronic)
Emerging Issues in Family and Individual Resilience
ISBN 978-3-031-98936-0 ISBN 978-3-031-98937-7 (eBook)
https://doi.org/10.1007/978-3-031-98937-7

This Springer imprint is published by the registered company Springer Nature Switzerland AG
The registered company address is: Gewerbestrasse 11, 6330 Cham, Switzerland

To the parents, caregivers, and communities who foster resilience in the face of adversity. To the practitioners and researchers dedicated to bridging knowledge and practice for the well-being of children and families. And to all those working to create a healthier, more inclusive future—this book is for you.

Preface

Food and nutrition are fundamental physiological needs, but they extend beyond providing emotional, social, and cultural connection along with experiences of joy and pleasure. Our interactions with food and health are deeply shaped by our experiences, environments, and relationships. Stress, adversity, and resilience influence not only what we eat but also how we engage with food, our bodies, and those around us. *Stress, Resilience, and Healthy Relationships with Food and Family* brings together research, practice, and lived experiences to explore these complex dynamics.

This book emerged from the Center for Family Resilience's yearlong research-to-practice speaker series, designed to bridge the gap between academic research and real-world practice. Throughout the series, experts from diverse fields—including nutrition, psychology, medicine, and family science—examined the ways in which early life experiences, food environments, and sociocultural factors shape eating behaviors and health outcomes. The series culminated in a conference where scholars, practitioners, and community members engaged in rich discussions, many of which informed the chapters in this volume.

The book covers a range of critical topics, from the interplay between adverse and protective childhood experiences (ACEs and PACEs) and food behaviors, to the role of epigenetics in obesity risk, to the ways in which parents seek and apply nutrition information for their children. It also explores food environments, resilience in gender-diverse populations, and strategies for fostering healthier eating habits. In terms of the Family Resilience Model (Henry et al., 2015), multiple Family Adaptive Systems (FAS) are represented, including the Maintenance FAS (Chaps. 1, 3, 4, and 6), the Emotion FAS (Chaps. 3, 4, 5, and 6), the Control FAS (Chaps. 2, 3, 4, and 6), the Meaning FAS (Chap. 5), and the Stress Response FAS (Chaps. 1 and 4). Throughout, the voices of parents and caregivers provide essential perspectives, grounding research in lived experiences.

Designed for academics, students, practitioners, and policymakers, this book offers both evidence-based insights and practical applications for those working to support healthier relationships with food and family. We hope that it inspires further dialogue, research, and action toward a future where individuals and communities can thrive.

Stillwater, OK, USA

Ginger Welch
Amanda W. Harrist
Haley Hall

Reference

Henry, C. S., Morris, A. S., & Harrist, A. W. (2015). Family resilience: Moving into the third wave. *Family Relations*, *64*(1), 22–43. https://doi.org/10.1111/fare.12106

Acknowledgments

This book is the result of a collaborative effort, and we are deeply grateful to those who contributed their time, expertise, and insights to bring it to fruition.

The voices of parents who have supported their children's resilience in the face of food- and body-related challenges are highlighted in the Breakout Boxes accompanying the chapters. We are grateful for the insights provided by these parents, including M. Decker, Crystal Kite, Kaitlin Lumen, Sonia Manjarrez, and Briana Riggs. We are also grateful to the following Oklahoma State University Honors College students who listened to these parents and shared their stories: Erin Barnard, Delaney Beak, Rylan Burrows, Madalyn Cory, Reagan Decker, Lily Downing, Allie Dreyer, Addie Galante, James Hinds, Hadley Keith, Maddie Kenney, Emily Lair, Bella Panganiban, Emma Phelps, Kaitlyn Rose, Emma-Frances Smith, Raylee Stuckey, Jackson Wallace, Keeley Warder, and Laci Wood.

We appreciate the thoughtful feedback provided by our reviewers: Hannah Appleseth, Erica Crockett-Barberea, Emily Doherty, Susette Moyers, and Brooke Tuttle.

And finally, we wish to acknowledge the incredible team at the Center for Family Resilience for organizing and hosting the research-to-practice seminar series that laid the foundation for this book. In particular, we are grateful to Brooke Tuttle, the director, and Hannah Alsabrook, program manager, for their leadership and dedication to this project. We also extend our thanks to the Pediatric Obesity Extension for Community Healthcare Outcomes (ECHO) for their support in bringing speakers and participants together from the seminar series. Lastly, we are especially appreciative to Dr. Colony Fugate for her support from this project's beginning to end.

Contents

About the Editors and Contributors

About the Editors

Haley Hall is a registered dietitian specializing in pediatric nutrition, with a focus on children who have experienced adversity. She works in private practice and serves as the registered dietitian for the Pediatric Obesity ECHO program. Currently, she is pursuing a doctoral degree in Human Development and Family Science at Oklahoma State University, where she is a research assistant for the Center for Family Resilience. Her research focuses on biopsychosocial factors that impact pediatric nutrition.

Amanda W. Harrist is an emeritus professor of human development and family science at Oklahoma State University. She was an Associate Director for Community Outreach for the OSU Center for Family Resilience for 13 years and an Administrative Core member, Center for Integrative Research on Childhood Adversity, and NIH COBRE center for 6 years. Her research centers on the family and peer contexts of development of children's social competence and maladjustment, particularly as exhibited in preschool and the early years of school. She and colleagues have developed a Family Resilience Model, and she has been series editor or editor for the Volumes 1–7 in the *Emerging issues in family and individual resilience* book series.

Ginger Welch is a clinical professor of human development and family science at Oklahoma State University where her work is focused on community outreach. She is an Associate Director for Community Outreach for the OSU Center for Family Resilience, and a pediatric psychologist on the Pediatric Obesity ECHO program. Her research interests include early childhood mental health and maternal and child health. She is an editor of a previous family resilience volume.

Contributors

Sebastian M. Barr, Ph.D. (he/him), is a counseling psychologist who works as a psychotherapist, researcher, consultant, and educator. He has contributed to multiple academic and clinical texts on affirming and trauma-informed psychotherapy with members of the trans community and serves on the editorial board of *Psychotherapy and Psychology of Sexual Orientation and Gender Diversity*. Dr. Barr's research has been recognized by awards from the World Professional Association for Trans Health and the American Psychological Association's Society for the Psychology of Sexual Orientation and Gender Diversity. He was the 2023 recipient of the Early Career Clinical Practice Award from the Society for Counseling Psychology and is a past scholar-in-residence at Faberllull in Olot, Catalonia/Spain. Dr. Barr is a proud trans man and incorporates personal and community perspectives in his work as appropriate.

Lana Beasley, Ph.D., is a Professor of Psychiatry and Behavioral Sciences at the Center for Health Sciences at Oklahoma State University. She is also the Director of Resilience, Adversity, and Interventions at the Center for Integrative Research on Childhood Adversity.

Ashlea Braun, Ph.D., R.D. (she/her/hers), is an Assistant Professor of Health Promotion Sciences in the Hudson College of Public Health and Tobacco Settlement Endowment Trust Health Promotion Research Center at the OU Health Stephenson Cancer Center at University of Oklahoma Health Sciences. Her research is focused on understanding and testing ways in which individuals can be supported to improve diet in the context of challenging sociocultural environments. She commonly includes autonomy-supportive approaches, such as motivational interviewing, and is a member of the Motivational Interviewing Network of Trainers. As a registered dietitian, she is also interested in behavioral effects of specific foods and food components and how these can support, or hinder, behavior change efforts with a particular emphasis on cancer prevention and control.

Timothy R. Brick, Ph.D., is an Associate Professor of Human Development and Family Studies at Penn State University, University Park, PA. Brick completed his Ph.D. in Cognitive and Quantitative Psychology at the University of Virginia. In his research program, Brick explores how human interactions and internal experiences influence behavior, focusing on complex contexts like parenting, education, recovery, aging, and neurodiversity. He develops and deploys innovative methods for capturing data in real time, such as wearable GPS sensors, heart rate monitors, and smartphone-based ecological momentary assessment (EMA) surveys. He also specializes in advanced data analytic techniques, including machine learning and privacy-preserving approaches. By creating new tools for data collection and analysis, Brick aims to build more effective and ethical approaches to research in the behavioral and health sciences.

Haley Hall, M.S., R.D./L.D., is a pediatric registered dietitian and a PhD candidate in Human Development and Family Science at Oklahoma State University. She earned her M.S. in Nutritional Sciences from Oklahoma State University. Her work with families and research focuses on promoting family resilience and well-being.

Jennifer Hays-Grudo, Ph.D., is a Regents Professor of Psychiatry and Behavioral Sciences at the Center for Health Sciences at Oklahoma State University. She is also the project director at the Center for Integrative Research on Childhood Adversity.

Allison Doub Hepworth, Ph.D., R.D., is an Assistant Professor of Nutritional Sciences at Oklahoma State University, Stillwater, OK and a registered dietitian. She completed her Ph.D. at Penn State University, University Park, PA in Human Development and Family Studies with minors in Information Sciences and Technology and Nutritional Sciences. She then completed a postdoctoral fellowship in early childhood prevention research at the University of Maryland School of Social Work, Baltimore, MD. Hepworth's research program focuses on how technology use and information seeking behaviors influence what and how parents feed their children and adult eating behavior. She aims to help individuals develop nutritious and satisfying eating patterns within the broader context of family and social systems.

Jillian M. Joyce, Ph.D., R.D., is a Registered Dietitian who hates kale and loves chocolate, Associate Professor, and Co-director of the Tactical Fitness and Nutrition Lab at Oklahoma State University. She is originally from Pittsburgh, PA, and after graduation, spent 9 years moving around the country with her husband for his active-duty Army service working in a variety of settings as a dietitian. As a researcher, Jill investigates how healthy tactical athletes (fire, law enforcement, military) eat, why they eat the way they do, and effective interventions to help them fuel properly for health and performance.

Douglas Knutson, Ph.D., L.H.S.P., A.B.P.P. (he/him), is the Myron Ledbetter/Bob Lemon Counseling Psychology Diversity Associate Professor and Director of Training for the Counseling Psychology Doctoral Program at Oklahoma State University. He is a licensed health service psychologist, board certified in counseling psychology. Dr. Knutson coordinates the Health, Education, and Rural Empowerment Lab, the 2022 recipient of the AMSA/GLMA LGBTQ Health Achievement Award. He serves on the American Psychological Association (APA) Committee on Rural Health and as an associate editor for the Journal of Rural Mental Health. He was the 2023 recipient of the APA Excellence in Rural Psychology Award and the 2023 Judy E. Hall Early Career Psychologist Award from the National Register of Health Service Psychologists. In addition to a broad range of articles and book chapters, Dr. Knutson is co-author of the book, *Counseling in a Gender Expansive World: Resources to Support Therapeutic Practice*.

Kristen McClanahan, M.S., R.D., is a clinical dietitian based in Tulsa, Oklahoma. Born and raised in the state, she believes everyone should experience Braum's ice cream at least once in their lifetime. Kristen's research has focused on the role of the environment in dietary habits. She believes everyone deserves a nutritious diet that fuels both body and soul.

Carolina Quijada, B.S., is a third-year medical student at Oklahoma State University College of Medicine with a strong commitment to serving underserved communities, particularly in the Hispanic/Latino community. She received her Bachelor of Science in Human Nutrition from Oklahoma State University. Carolina has conducted research on Adverse Childhood Experiences (ACEs) under the mentorship of Dr. Dolores Vazquez-Sanroman, focusing on the long-term health impacts of childhood trauma. Carolina's work is driven by personal experience and the passion to mitigate health disparities for underserved communities in Oklahoma.

Pamela Gonzalez Sanchez, M.S., is a doctoral student and a member of the Oklahoma State University Tactical Fitness and Nutrition lab. She is originally from Mexico and pursued her undergraduate degree in biochemistry. Then, she switched gears to clinical nutrition for her master's degree. After 2 years of independent practice as a dietitian, Pamela moved abroad and joined Oklahoma State University in 2021. Her research focuses on tactical athletes' families, including firefighters, law enforcement, and military personnel. She dives deep into understanding the current eating habits of children and spouses and aims to develop effective interventions to improve these families' overall health and well-being.

Meg L. Small, Ph.D., is the Director for Social Impact at the Edna Bennett Pierce Prevention Research Center and Associate Research Professor of Human Development and Family Studies at Penn State University, University Park, PA. She also serves as the Academic Director of the Impact Incubator within the Evidence-to-Impact Collaborative at Penn State University. Small completed her Ph.D. in Public and Community Health at the University of Maryland. As an expert in prevention research and entrepreneurial methods, Small thrives as a collaborator and catalyst, bringing together ideas, people, and resources to amplify the reach of research-driven solutions. Committed to closing the gap between discovery and impact, she partners with interdisciplinary colleagues to translate evidence into scalable, real-world impact.

Bek Urban, M.A. (they/any), is a PhD Candidate in counseling psychology at Oklahoma State University and an incoming Postdoctoral Research Fellow at Virginia Commonwealth University. Bek's research is broadly concerned with queer health and health equity with a specific focus on risk and maintenance factors for eating disorders among transgender and gender-diverse individuals. Bek is the chair of the Mentoring Committee for the Society for the Psychology of Sexual Orientation and Gender Diversity within the American Psychological Association (APA). Bek is also active in APA's Society for Counseling Psychology and American

Psychological Association of Graduate Students. In 2024, Bek was the recipient of the Society for Counseling Psychology's Counseling Health Psychology Student Research Award and was named the Outstanding Graduate Student for the Society for the Advancement of Sexual Orientation and Gender Diversity.

Dolores Vazquez-Sanroman, Ph.D. (she/her/ella/suya), is an Associate Professor in the Department of Anatomy and Cell Biology at the Oklahoma State University Center for Health Sciences and a substance abuse researcher. Her research focuses on understanding the effects of early life stress and drug abuse using an animal model of addiction. She is interested in establishing a collaborative-translational research pipeline for securing funding to evaluate changes in circulating neurotrophins in opioid abuse patients. Dr. Vazquez received her Ph.D. degree in Psychology from the University of Jaime I in Valencia, Spain. Later, as a Postdoctoral Fellow in the Center for Drug Abuse Research Translation (CDART), funded by the National Institute on Drug Abuse at the University of Kentucky, I contributed to and validated a mood-based impulsivity model in rats under different housing conditions, with translational applications in human impulsivity disorders and adverse childhood traits. Today, her research focuses on the effects of neuronal plasticity and neurotrophic factors, particularly the brain-derived neurotrophic factor (BDNF). At this transitional point in her career, she developed an interest in understanding the effects of opioids on the gut-brain axis in adolescents, most importantly, the role of BNDF in microbiome opioid-induced dysbiosis.

Jason Zabel, B.S., is a fourth-year medical student at Oklahoma State University College of Osteopathic Medicine in Tulsa, Oklahoma. He earned his Bachelor of Science in biomedical sciences at Liberty University in Lynchburg, Virginia, with minors in both psychology and chemistry. Raised with strong Christian values, Jason deeply desires to share the love of Christ with all of his future patients through his career in medicine and is passionate about ensuring each person he interacts with feels valued and heard.

Olivia Zabel, B.S., is a fourth-year medical student at Oklahoma State University College of Osteopathic Medicine. She received her Bachelor of Science in Biomedical Sciences at Liberty University. With both of her parents working in the medical field, Olivia developed a passion for pursuing a career in family medicine from a young age. Through thoughtful community engagement and her strong faith in Jesus Christ, Olivia strives to medically serve others in all walks of life.

Chapter 1
ACEs and PACEs: Understanding and Changing the Dynamic Interplay of Food, Family, and Stress

Haley Hall, Lana Beasley, and Jennifer Hays-Grudo

Adverse childhood experiences (ACEs) is a term that refers to a set of potentially traumatic events or experiences that some individuals may face during childhood (Centers for Disease Control and Prevention [CDC], 2021). ACEs are prevalent and have potential negative impacts on mental and physical health (Anda et al., 2006; Felitti et al., 1998). Research is also clear that many individuals are able to adapt positively following significant adversity, a concept known as *resilience* (Luthar et al., 2000; Masten, 2001). Decades of research on resilience substantiate the importance of protective and compensatory experiences (PACEs) being present in children's lives (Hays-Grudo & Morris, 2020). These experiences include resources and relationships that can act as a buffer against the negative effects of adversity. In this chapter, we focus on understanding the relation between food, family, and stress by incorporating current research on nutrition, early adversity, and protective factors.

While there is a well-established understanding of how chronic stress impacts the developing nervous, endocrine, and immune systems (Danese & McEwen, 2012), less attention has been given to its effects on the metabolic system (Miller et al., 2011). Early life adversity triggers physiological stress responses resulting in the release of glucocorticoids and other stress hormones (Herman et al., 2016). This response affects the metabolic system through alterations in hormonal systems, disturbances to the gut microbiome, epigenetic modifications, and ultimately manifests as profound biobehavioral adaptations. Over time, these adaptations can lead to a decrease in healthy eating habits and an increase in maladaptive eating habits, such

H. Hall (✉)
Oklahoma State University, Stillwater, OK, USA
e-mail: haley.billings@okstate.edu

L. Beasley · J. Hays-Grudo
Oklahoma State University Center for Health Sciences, Tulsa, OK, USA

G. Welch et al. (eds.), *Stress, Resilience, and Healthy Relationships with Food and Family*, Emerging Issues in Family and Individual Resilience,
https://doi.org/10.1007/978-3-031-98937-7_1

as disordered eating, ultimately increasing the risk of developing a variety of nutrition-related chronic diseases.

Just as adversity and nutrition interact, so do protective factors and nutrition. Providing a safe and clean home with enough food helps create a health-promoting environment and reduces the impact of food insecurity. Incorporating family meals can serve as a source of rules and routines that promote predictability and provide time for social connection. Furthermore, the involvement of the broader community, such as the school system, can bridge the gap through programs and resources which can ensure equitable access to food, fostering both family and community resilience. This chapter emphasizes the holistic role of food and nutrition, extending beyond its primary function of fulfilling a basic physiological need, highlighting how it can act to bolster relationships, strengthen communities, and mitigate the consequences of adversity.

1.1 Adverse Childhood Experiences (ACEs)

1.1.1 Early Adversity

Adversity experienced during early childhood, such as various stressors, challenges, or traumatic experiences that a family may encounter, can have a significant impact on a child's development. These experiences can encompass a wide range of events including poverty, parental separation, exposure to violence, or other forms of family chaos and instability. The impact of adversity on early childhood development can be far reaching with symptoms manifesting in numerous ways across the lifespan. Early childhood is characterized by developmentally sensitive periods, which can influence an individual's response to adversity. Sensitive periods refer to specific windows of time when a child's brain is particularly vulnerable to certain types of environmental experiences (Knudsen, 2004). When adverse experiences disrupt these periods, they can negatively impact healthy physical, cognitive, emotional, and social development.

Childhood adversity is often captured through measures of adverse childhood experiences, or ACEs. The concept of ACEs was first studied and defined by researchers at the Centers for Disease Control and Prevention (CDC) and obesity specialists at Kaiser Permanente in the 1990s. The original ACEs study identified ten categories of childhood adversity that were significantly linked to physical and mental health problems as well as health-harming behaviors. The ten categories include physical, sexual, and emotional abuse, physical and emotional neglect, parental mental illness, substance abuse, criminality, domestic violence, and divorce or separation during the first 18 years of life (Felitti et al., 1998). Research using the ACEs framework has shown that experiencing multiple ACEs can increase the risk of various physical and mental health problems in adulthood, including heart disease, cancer, depression, substance abuse, and other chronic health conditions. The more ACEs an individual has experienced, the greater the risk of these negative outcomes (Felitti et al., 1998). Within the United States, it is estimated that around 58% of adults have experienced at least one ACE, and about 22% have experienced three or more ACEs (Giano et al., 2020).

1.1.2 Impact of Stress and Adversity

As stated previously, stress and adversity can have profound and wide-ranging impacts on individuals, in terms of physical and mental health, as well as overall well-being (Felitti et al., 1998). These effects can vary in intensity and duration depending on the individual, the specific circumstances, and the resources available to cope with these challenges. Prolonged exposure to stress and adversity has been linked to an increased risk of developing a myriad of chronic diseases like diabetes and certain cancers, partially explained by negative health behaviors (Felitti et al., 1998).

Chronic and acute stress stimulates the hypothalamic–pituitary–adrenal (HPA) axis to release glucocorticoids, such as cortisol (Herman et al., 2016) which signals a cascading effect that can lead to neuroendocrine responses, immunologic reactions, changes to brain structure and connectivity, and epigenetic changes. This cumulative dysregulation or "wear and tear" on the body is often referred to as allostatic load (McEwen, 1998). Changes in the HPA-axis can lead to undesirable outcomes such as cardiovascular issues, a compromised immune system, weight fluctuations, gastrointestinal problems, and sleep disturbances. In addition to physical health outcomes, early life stress can impact mental health outcomes. For example, early life stress can trigger or exacerbate anxiety disorders (McLaughlin & Hatzenbuehler, 2009; Pizzagalli, 2014), and exposure to extreme adversity may result in symptoms of Post-Traumatic Stress Disorder (McLaughlin et al., 2017).

Lastly, research has established a clear relationship between early life adversity, poor health behaviors, and negative outcomes across the lifespan. Experiencing even one of the ten original ACEs is associated with higher odds of tobacco use, alcohol problems, risky sexual behavior, poor self-reported health and quality of life, low exercise, and other psychosocial and behavioral outcomes compared to those with no ACEs (Petruccelli et al., 2019). This relationship intensifies for individuals who experienced more than one ACE. It is no surprise that higher cumulative levels of adversity are associated with increased odds of obesity, ischemic heart disease, cancer, stroke, diabetes, gastrointestinal disease, sleep disturbances, and respiratory disease among other health outcomes (Felitti et al., 1998; Petruccelli et al., 2019).

It is important to note that an individual's response to adversity is often adaptive in nature. The body is responsive to its environment and will modify physiological processes for efficiency and survival. However, the body functions as a system, so a change may be adaptive in some ways, but detrimental in others. This may be especially true for changes that occur during sensitive periods, or key developmental stages. Overall, the relationship between adverse experiences and health outcomes is complex (Hays-Grudo et al., 2021). Understanding ACEs is crucial for policy-makers, healthcare professionals, parents, educators, and communities due to the importance of early intervention, trauma-informed care, and support systems to help individuals who have experienced ACEs. Recognizing and addressing ACEs can be instrumental in preventing the long-term consequences of childhood trauma while promoting resiliency through understanding protective and compensatory experiences.

1.2 Protective and Compensatory Experiences (PACES)

Protective factors are characteristics, attributes, or circumstances that can help individuals, families, and communities to cope with and thrive in the face of adversity or stressful situations (Walsh, 2003). Based on a review of decades of research on resilience, Hays-Grudo and Morris (2020) identified ten experiences that help children overcome adverse circumstances and promote positive well-being. These ten Protective and Compensatory Childhood Experiences (PACEs) may act as a buffer to ACEs by providing children and youth with two broad categories of protection: supportive relationships and environmental conditions and resources that promote development (Hays-Grudo & Morris, 2020). Supportive relationships refer to the presence of caring and nurturing individuals in a child's life. These individuals can be parents, caregivers, teachers, mentors, or any positive influence which provides emotional support, guidance, and a sense of security. Supportive relationships can act as a protective factor by helping children cope with stress and adversity. They can provide a safe emotional space for children to express their feelings and seek help when needed. Developmental conditions and resources include the physical, social, and educational aspects of a child's surroundings that promote cognitive, social, and emotional development. They include having basic physical needs met, along with opportunities to learn, grow and develop skills. An enriching environment can compensate for deficits and foster development, even in the face of adversity. Each of the 10 PACEs is described in more detail in the following section (Table 1.1).

1.2.1 Unconditional Love

Children need to feel loved and know they are cared about. Decades of attachment research highlight how important unconditional love is for a child (Darling Rasmussen et al., 2019; Flaherty & Sadler, 2011; Schore, 2001; Simmons et al., 2009). Unconditional love, which is often accompanied by warmth and nurturance, can lead to secure attachment between a child and a caregiver. Feeling safe and

Table 1.1 Protective and compensatory experiences

When you were growing up, prior to your 18th birthday:		
1. Did you have someone who loved you unconditionally (you did not doubt that they cared about you)?	YES	NO
2. Did you have at least one best friend (someone you could trust, had fun with)?	YES	NO
3. Did you do anything regularly to help others (e.g., volunteer at a hospital, nursing home, church) or do special projects in the community to help others (food drives, habitat for humanity)?	YES	NO
4. Were you regularly involved in organized sports groups (e.g., soccer, basketball, track) or other physical activity (e.g., competitive cheer, gymnastics, dance, marching band)?	YES	NO
5. Were you an active member of at least one civic group or a non-sport social group such as scouts, religious group, or youth group?	YES	NO
6. Did you have an engaging hobby—An artistic/creative or intellectual pastime either alone or in a group (e.g., chess club, debate team, musical instrument or vocal group, theater, spelling bee, or did you read a lot)?	YES	NO
7. Was there an adult (not your parent) you trusted and could count on when you needed help or advice (e.g., coach, teacher, minister, neighbor, relative)?	YES	NO
8. Was your home typically clean and safe with enough food to eat?	YES	NO
9. Overall, did your schools provide the resources and academic experiences you needed to learn?	YES	NO
10. In your home, were there rules that were clear and fairly administered?	YES	NO

secure allows the child to explore and be curious about their environment, develop a positive self-view, and learn to trust others (Bowlby, 1982).

1.2.2 Having a Best Friend

Having a best friend can help mitigate some of the negative impacts of childhood adversity. Adolescents who report higher levels of friendship had better psychosocial outcomes during adolescence and young adulthood (Van Harmelen et al., 2017). Friendship is an important protective factor throughout the entire life course. For example, adults who experienced high ACEs but also reported high levels of social support had lower risks of depression than those who did not have high levels of social support (Von Cheong et al., 2017).

1.2.3 Having a Mentor

Caring and trusted adults outside of the immediate family can play an essential role in child development. Trustworthy adults, such as coaches, teachers, grandparents, or other relatives, can provide support, advice, and comfort when caregivers may not be available. Mentors can teach moral values, foster self-esteem, promote positive behavior outcomes, and support mental health (Southwick et al., 2007).

1.2.4 Being a Part of a Group

Membership in a group can foster a sense of belonging in the community. Additionally, group membership helps foster identity development, and aid children in developing their own values and morals. Being part of a group can lead to a sense of belonging which is associated with more positive behavioral outcomes for adolescence (Newman et al., 2007). Not only does belonging to a group provide social and behavioral benefits, but it can also promote resilience through physiological pathways. For example, a study in one indigenous community found that higher levels of belonging reduced the interaction between ACEs and inflammation (John-Henderson et al., 2020).

1.2.5 Volunteering

Volunteering and helping others can provide children with a sense of connection to the larger community, foster empathy, and promote perspective taking. Volunteering is also associated with positive mental health, physical health, life satisfaction, and social well-being (Yeung et al., 2018).

1.2.6 Physical Activity

Being physically active is important for health and can help children regulate the physiological effects of stress. Organized sports can provide connection with other children and other adults. Participating in team sports allows a child to develop a number of skills including goal setting, self-regulation, and self-esteem. For adults, physical activity has been shown to mediate the relationship between ACEs and depression (Boisgontier et al., 2020) and is associated with improved health-related quality of life (Moon & Han, 2022). Additionally, physical activity has been found to reduce the effects of ACEs and depression on activities of daily living (Boisgontier et al., 2020).

1.2.7 Having a Hobby

Hobbies can include activities such as dance, photography, cooking, chess, writing, and many other activities. Hobbies can teach discipline, perseverance, self-regulation, and patience in the context of fun (Steinberg & Simon, 2019). Hobbies can provide an outlet for creative expression and identity exploration and can foster a sense of mastery, competence, and self-esteem (Mahoney et al., 2003).

1.2.8 Clean, Safe Home with Enough Food

To create a nurturing environment, a home should be safe and clean with enough food to eat. Adequate shelter and food supply are basic physiological needs which must be met before safety and security, love and belonging, and self-esteem (Maslow, 1943). Research has found that children who live in homes that are cluttered and unclean have worse outcomes as compared to children living in clean homes, even when things like parenting and resources are equal (Vernon-Feagans et al., 2016).

1.2.9 Rules and Routines

Fair rules and predictable routines create a sense of safety and predictability (Harrist et al., 2019). During early childhood, family routines create opportunities for social interactions which can lead to vocabulary enrichment, social skill development, and academic achievement (Spagnola & Fiese, 2007). Adolescents whose parents monitor their friends and activities are less likely to engage in risky behaviors and have better school performance (Affuso et al., 2016; Dittus et al., 2023). As children grow older, it is important for them to have input into their rules.

1.2.10 Opportunity to Learn

Children require opportunities to learn through high-quality education. Education is a crucial component of child development with quality early childhood education showing a seven to one return on investment related to positive child outcomes (Heckman, 2012). Attending a school that provides the resources and opportunities to have positive academic experiences helps children facilitate mastery of knowledge (Card & Krueger, 1998). Additionally, when children attend a high-quality school, they are often among peers who do well in schools and families who value education. Being among such peers amplifies students' performance, as students tend to fall or rise in performance, based on those around them. Evidence across many disciplines (psychology, economics, and sociology) finds that high-quality education is one of the best predictors of later life success and happiness (Assari, 2019; Diener et al., 1999; Stryzhak, 2020).

Overall, protective and compensatory experiences act as buffers against the negative impact of adverse experiences and can contribute to resilience and well-being. Protective experiences can lead to positive developmental outcomes and can help mitigate the negative consequences associated with ACEs. These relationships and resources are essential during childhood but are protective at all stages across the lifespan. It is also important to think of key protective factors through a broader lens such as nutrition. Specifically, nutrition is a fundamental component when thinking of adversity as it can act as a risk or protective factor in numerous ways.

1.3 Adversity Through a Nutritional Lens

1.3.1 Neurobiological Adaptations

Adversity, particularly chronic stress, and traumatic experiences can have a significant impact on the metabolic system. The body's metabolic processes are tightly interconnected with the endocrine and nervous systems, and disruptions in these systems can lead to various metabolic changes. While the impact of chronic stress on the nervous, endocrine, and immune systems is well understood (Danese & McEwen, 2012), less attention has been given to its effects on the metabolic system.

Chronic stress activates the HPA-axis, which results in the stimulation of glucocorticoids (Herman et al., 2016). In addition to their role in stress response, glucocorticoids function as a key regulator of metabolic homeostasis. When the body encounters stress, it releases glucose and free fatty acids to provide quick energy, which can be helpful in an emergency. This "fight or flight" response, while advantageous in a real or perceived threat, can be damaging following prolonged activation. Continuous or frequent stress responses can lead to negative long-term consequences due to changes in metabolic risk markers, such as cholesterol levels, glucose metabolism, and body composition (Akalestou et al., 2020; Suvarna et al., 2020).

In addition to its critical role in stress adaptation, the hypothalamus also aids in the regulation of hunger and satiety hormones (Wren & Bloom, 2007). These hormones control energy stores, regulate body weight, pace gastric emptying, and control appetite (Wren & Bloom, 2007). It is suggested that early life adversity interferes with the expression, regulation, and interaction of these hormones. For example, research has shown that childhood adversity can lead to changes in satiety hormones like leptin and ghrelin. Alterations in leptin, responsible for promoting satiety, can result in increased food enjoyment, responsiveness, fussiness, and satiety in young children who have experienced early adversity (de Lima et al., 2022). Ghrelin, often referred to as the "hunger" hormone, helps regulate appetite and body weight through glucose homeostasis and lipid metabolism (Ibrahim Abdalla, 2015). Daniels et al. (2023) found that history of early life adversity in young adults was associated with lower fasted ghrelin levels compared to controls, even when BMI, age, and sex were controlled for. Beyond its role in appetite regulation and energy metabolism, ghrelin functions in gastric acid secretion, bone health via osteoblast regulation, learning and memory, sleep patterns, aging, and as a protective hormone in neurodegenerative disease (Ibrahim Abdalla, 2015). Taken all together, these findings suggest a potential mechanism to connect early life adversity to a range of negative outcomes, although more research is needed.

Childhood stress and adversity can alter the gut microbiome which, among other things, plays a role in digestion and metabolism. The gut microbiome comprises microbiota and their byproducts that inhabit the gastrointestinal tract (Hantsoo & Zemel, 2021) and play critical roles in metabolizing and absorbing nutrients and drugs, producing essential vitamins, regulating the immune system, serving as an epithelial barrier, and producing neurotransmitters (Cho & Blaser, 2012). Beyond the gastrointestinal tract, the gut microbiota interacts with the brain and central nervous system through bi-directional communication pathways known as the gut-brain axis (Hantsoo & Zemel, 2021). Stress and adversity can lead to changes in the composition and diversity of the gut microbiome, which may affect various aspects of health and well-being. For example, one study found differences in composition and diversity within the microbiome of adolescents institutionalized in orphanages compared with a control group (Reid et al., 2021).

Lastly, childhood adversity can lead to altered gene expression through epigenetic changes (Parade et al., 2021). Epigenetic changes refer to modifications that influence gene expression without altering the DNA sequence (see Meaney, 2010, for review). In this way, ACEs can change the way that genes are transcribed and expressed. For example, brain-derived neurotrophic factor (BDNF) plays a critical role in synaptic plasticity and memory, neural differentiation throughout development, and regulation of excitatory and inhibitory synaptic processes during adulthood (Miranda et al., 2019). Research in mice models documents epigenetic changes in BDNF as a result of early life adversity (Roth & Sweatt, 2011). Maniam and Morris (2010) found that access to a high fat diet reduced anxiety and depression like behaviors and normalized BDNF alterations for rat pups that were postnatally separated from dams. Although these studies have not yet been replicated in humans, they suggest that dietary patterns may play a role in genetic and behavioral changes after early life adversity.

1.3.2 *Executive Function, Emotion Regulation, and Impulse Control*

Childhood adversity can alter the structure and function of the prefrontal cortex, the brain region responsible for cognitive functioning (Teicher et al., 2016; van der Kolk, 2003). These changes can lead to difficulties in decision-making, executive functioning, emotion regulation, and impulse control. These alterations have a direct impact on health and nutrition-related behaviors. For example, research suggests that children who experience chronic stress may turn to emotional eating as a way to cope with stress and counteract the effects of the body's stress response system (Kazmierski et al., 2022). As mentioned earlier, glucocorticoids are released in response to a stressor, which is associated with emotional eating, or a drive to consume "comfort foods" typically high in sugar, fat, and total calories. While this may provide short-term regulation, relying on this coping mechanism consistently can result in a positive energy balance, unhealthy eating patterns, and long-term health consequences (Kazmierski et al., 2022). Furthermore, stress and adversity can diminish dopaminergic responses, potentially leading to an increased tendency for reward-seeking behavior, including emotional eating. These effects may be more pronounced in individuals who already struggle with emotion regulation. For example, young adults who experience polyvictimization and higher levels of emotional dysregulation reported the highest levels of disordered eating (Hasselle et al., 2017).

1.3.3 *Biobehavioral Adaptations*

Chronic activation of the stress response system can trigger biobehavioral adaptations. For example, turning to food as a means of coping with stress can lead to long-term changes in eating habits. Yoon and colleagues found that cumulative ACE scores were correlated with an increase in maladaptive eating behaviors, such as overeating and binge eating, and a decrease in healthy or adaptive eating behaviors, such as intuitive eating and mindful eating (Yoon et al., 2022). Ultimately, these long-term adaptations can lead to serious consequences including elevated risk of eating disorders, obesity, heart disease, cancer, depression, substance abuse, and other chronic health conditions.

1.4 Resilience Through a Nutritional Lens

1.4.1 Nutrition as a Protective Factor

There is an interplay between family, food, and stress. This section will focus on the interplay between family and food and how nutrition can serve as a protective factor. PACEs include two important protective domains: supportive relationships and an enriching environment (Hays-Grudo & Morris, 2020). Nutrition plays an essential role in both domains and is therefore an important component to consider (Table 1.2).

1.4.2 Nutrition and Supportive Relationships

Food is an inherently social component of life, often serving as a context for shared experiences. During infancy, feeding provide opportunity for caregivers to bond with their child. During these moments, caregivers learn to intuitively respond to the infant's cues and the infant learns to trust their caregivers. These shared moments are not only essential for fulfilling the child's nutritional needs, but also for nurturing a sense of safety and predictability (Satter, 1990). Additionally, these early interactions allow a child to learn to communicate needs and desires, explore new foods, develop fine motor skills, and experience mastery (Black & Aboud, 2011). As infants transition to toddlerhood, family meals are often a context in which they practice their autonomy (Satter, 1995). As toddlers develop into children and eventually adolescents, meals extend beyond the immediate family to include peers and

Table 1.2 PACEs, nutrition PACEs, and benefits

PACE	Nutrition PACE	Benefits
Unconditional love	Shared meals	• Opportunity for bonding and connection • Age-appropriate skill development • Social interaction with family, peers, and community
Having a clean and safe home with enough food	Food security	• Improved behavioral, academic, and emotional development
Family routines and rituals	Regular family meals	• Parent/caregiver modeling • Healthier eating patterns • Maintenance of a healthy weight • Higher self-esteem • Better mental health outcomes • Higher levels of family togetherness
Access to quality school	Free and reduced school meals	• Reduced food insufficiency • Better overall dietary quality • Improved academic outcomes • Increased school attendance rates

others within the neighborhood, school, and community. This shared experience persists into adulthood, where meals become a means to connect with family, peers, coworkers, significant others, and others. Regardless of life stage, nutrition remains a basic human need that also functions as an opportunity to create and strengthen social connections.

1.4.3 Nutrition and Enriched Environments

Ensuring a clean and safe home with enough food to eat is an essential PACE. Food insecurity plays a pivotal role in the developmental trajectories of children, impacting their behavioral, academic, and emotional well-being from infancy through adolescence (Shankar et al., 2017). Recent statistics from 2021 reveal that 12.5% of households with children experienced food insecurity (United States Department of Agriculture, 2023). Moreover, there is a noteworthy correlation between higher ACE scores and an increased likelihood of encountering food insecurity (Jackson et al., 2019). To address this issue, federally funded programs such as the Supplemental Nutrition Assistance Program (SNAP), National School Lunch Program (NSLP), and Women, Infants, and Children (WIC) program have been instrumental in reducing food insecurity rates (Gundersen & Ziliak, 2015).

Incorporating family meals as part of a family's routine can serve as a protective factor with parents and caregivers playing a primary role in shaping children's dietary behaviors and habits. Shared mealtimes can provide a time for parents and caregivers to serve as role models for healthy eating (Mahmood et al., 2021). Children and adolescents who regularly consume meals with family members tend to establish healthier eating patterns, maintain a healthy weight, experience higher levels of self-esteem, have increased positive mental health outcomes, and share higher levels of family togetherness (Berge et al., 2018; Hammons & Fiese, 2011; Prior & Limbert, 2013; Spagnola & Fiese, 2007). Eating meals together as a family can benefit the physical and mental health of both children and caretakers and can promote higher levels of family functioning (Utter et al., 2018).

Breakout Box 1.1: A View from the Foster Care System
In my experience in working with children who have been exposed to Adverse Childhood Experiences (ACEs) as an Executive Director for CASA for Kids, I have noticed behaviors such as food hoarding and using food/eating as a way of control and feeling safe. These behaviors may be due to physical neglect resulting in food insecurity or having food used as a punishment within their environment. I have noticed throughout my time in working with these children that the two main aspects of reversing these negative food behaviors are time and consistency. Protective and Compensatory Experiences (PACEs) that can be used to assist time and consistency are nurturing relationships and

> enriched environments. These PACEs help to create a sense of belonging and validate children's experiences. Unconditional love is a critical part of children's development and life-long attachment styles and helps to build nurturing relationships with the child. Having an enriched environment includes talking about food health positively and allowing children to have a designated area where they can access food at all times. It is important to note that both of these aids improve the quality of life for these children. In my line of work, the ultimate goal is to reunite children with their biological families. One way that is used to safely reintegrate parents with their biological children includes a parenting class focusing on food and health safety. The most important thing to remember is that the child's health and safety comes first. At the end of the day, we will do what is best for the child and whatever we can to meet their needs effectively
>
> — Sarah Priest, Executive Director for CASA for Kids, Inc., an organization that recruit, train, and supervise Court Appointed Special Advocate (CASA) volunteers to advocate for and improve the well-being of children involved in the foster care system

Outside of the home, access to a quality school can provide exposure to protective factors beyond an education. Schools are often full of caring adults that can act as mentors with peers who can serve as friends. Schools also offer opportunities such as sports teams, clubs, and volunteer projects. Classrooms often thrive on structured rules and routines which can also serve as a protective factor for children. Lastly, schools offer access to beneficial programs such as the School Breakfast Program (SBP) and the National School Lunch Program (NSLP), which have been shown to reduce food insecurity by as much as 14% (Huang & Barnidge, 2016). Additionally, these food programs are associated with higher diet quality, improved academic outcomes, and increased attendance rates, particularly for at-risk children (Cohen et al., 2021).

1.5 Implications

1.5.1 Implications for Understanding Family Resilience

Understanding family resilience in the context of childhood adversity and its relationship with nutrition can have profound implications for various aspects of family life and well-being.

1. *Supportive Family Dynamics*: Recognizing the protective role of nutrition within the family can lead to a greater emphasis on creating supportive mealtime environments. Shared mealtimes can lead to conversations, increased connection,

improved emotional support, and an opportunity to teach children healthy eating habits. When families prioritize shared meals, they foster a sense of togetherness which can promote resilience in the face of adversity.

2. *Interdisciplinary Approach*: Understanding the relationship between family, food, and stress provides practitioners with multiple points of potential support to promote family resilience. It is essential that families have their basic needs met, which includes access to adequate healthy food. Practitioners should be aware of community resources that might help families meet these needs prior to focusing on other goals related to family resilience.

1.5.2 Implications for Practice and/or Policy

Practice and policy can foster family resilience by supporting programs and practices that increase equitable access to healthy and nutritious foods.

1. *Reduce Food Insecurity Through Programmatic Support*: Understanding the connection between nutrition and family resilience highlights the importance of ensuring all families have access to adequate, nutritious food. Policymakers and communities can work together to address food insecurity by supporting programs like the Supplemental Nutrition Assistance Program (SNAP), National Schools Lunch Program (NSLP), and Woman, Infants, and Children (WIC) program. This, in turn, can have a significant impact on the physical and mental health of children, families, and the community as a whole.
2. *Community Support*: Understanding family resilience in the context of nutrition extends beyond the family context. Communities can play a pivotal role in supporting families, especially in providing access to nutritious food and fostering social connections through shared meals and activities. By recognizing the positive impact of community initiatives, local organizations and institutions can work to create environments that promote resilience, emphasizing the importance of nutrition as a protective factor.

1.6 Conclusions and Future Directions

In conclusion, this book chapter provides a general overview of the relationship between childhood adversity, protective experiences, and nutrition. We highlight the multifaceted ways that ACEs impact physical, cognitive, emotional, and social development. We also discuss the physiological impact of chronic stress, particularly on the metabolic system. Chronic stress leads to adaptations that can result in physiological changes, maladaptive eating behaviors, and long-term health consequences. As such, recognizing the power and influence of food, supportive family dynamics, and effective stress management is essential.

Food and nutrition serve a purpose beyond nurturing our bodies. Adequate nutrition is not only a basic need but is also an integral protective factor. As parents, practitioners, community members, and policy makers, we must recognize the power and influence that access to quality nutrition has on all individuals and consider ways to create and support equitable access to mitigate the long-term consequences of childhood adversity. It is critical that we create a safe and clean home environment with enough food to eat and establish rules and routines related to mealtimes. As a community, families can lean into the social benefits of food and connect with one another at the table. We can promote family and community resilience through food banks and other resources to ensure everyone has access to enough food. Within our policies, it is critical that we address and minimize food insecurity through continued support and funding for programs such as SNAP, NSLP, and WIC. Recognizing the complex relationship between food, family, and stress, and the crucial role of nutrition in this dynamic, can ultimately lead to improved outcomes for individuals, families, and communities facing adversity.

Discussion Questions

1. The chapter highlights the complex interplay between childhood adversity, family resilience, and nutrition. How can an interdisciplinary approach help professionals better understand and address the impact of adversity on child development and the role of nutrition in fostering family resilience?
2. Current literature supports a wide range of negative health implications associated with childhood adversity. How can we use this knowledge to improve intervention and prevention strategies?
3. Nutrition-related PACEs can be supported at the family, community, and policy level. How can you promote these PACEs within the work that you do?
4. Nutrition is presented as a key protective factor within the family environment. Discuss other ways nutrition may serve a role in family and community resilience.

References

Affuso, G., Bacchini, D., & Miranda, M. C. (2016). The contribution of school-related parental monitoring, self-determination, and self-efficacy to academic achievement. *The Journal of Educational Research, 110*(5), 565–574. https://doi.org/10.1080/00220671.2016.1149795

Akalestou, E., Genser, L., & Rutter, G. A. (2020). Glucocorticoid metabolism in obesity and following weight loss. *Frontiers in Endocrinology, 11*, 59. https://doi.org/10.3389/fendo.2020.00059

Anda, R. F., Felitti, V. J., Bremner, J. D., Walker, J. D., Whitfield, C. H., Perry, B. D., Dube, S. R., & Giles, W. H. (2006). The enduring effects of abuse and related adverse experiences in childhood: A convergence of evidence from neurobiology and epidemiology. *European Archives of Psychiatry and Clinical Neuroscience, 256*, 174–186. https://doi.org/10.1007/s00406-005-0624-4

Assari, S. (2019). Race, education attainment, and happiness in the United States. *International Journal of Epidemiologic Research, 6*(2), 76–82. https://doi.org/10.15171/ijer.2019.14

Berge, J. M., Miller, J., Watts, A., Larson, N., Loth, K. A., & Neumark-Sztainer, D. (2018). Intergenerational transmission of family meal patterns from adolescence to parenthood: Longitudinal associations with parents' dietary intake, weight-related behaviours and psychosocial Well-being. *Public Health Nutrition, 21*(2), 299–308. https://doi.org/10.1017/S1368980017002270

Black, M. M., & Aboud, F. E. (2011). Responsive feeding is embedded in a theoretical framework of responsive parenting. *The Journal of Nutrition, 141*(3), 490–494. https://doi.org/10.3945/jn.110.129973

Boisgontier, M. P., Orsholits, D., von Arx, M., Sieber, S., Miller, M. W., Courvoisier, D., Iversen, M. D., Cullati, S., & Cheval, B. (2020). Adverse childhood experiences, depressive symptoms, functional dependence, and physical activity: A moderated mediation model. *Journal of Physical Activity and Health, 17*(8), 790–799. https://doi.org/10.1123/jpah.2019-0133

Bowlby, J. (1982). *Attachment and loss: Vol. I. Attachment*. Basic Books. (Original work published 1969).

Card, D., & Krueger, A. B. (1998). School resources and student outcomes. *The Annals of the American Academy of Political and Social Science, 559*(1), 39–53. https://doi.org/10.1177/0002716298559001004

Centers for Disease Control and Prevention. (2021). *CDC-Kaiser Ace*. Center for Disease Control and Prevention. https://www.cdc.gov/violenceprevention/aces/about.html

Cho, I., & Blaser, M. J. (2012). The human microbiome: At the interface of health and disease. *Nature Reviews Genetics, 13*(4), 260–270. https://doi.org/10.1038/nrg3182

Cohen, J. F., Hecht, A. A., McLoughlin, G. M., Turner, L., & Schwartz, M. B. (2021). Universal school meals and associations with student participation, attendance, academic performance, diet quality, food security, and body mass index: A systematic review. *Nutrients, 13*(3), 911. https://doi.org/10.3390/nu13030911

Danese, A., & McEwen, B. S. (2012). Adverse childhood experiences, allostasis, allostatic load, and age-related disease. *Physiology & Behavior, 106*(1), 29–39. https://doi.org/10.1016/j.physbeh.2011.08.019

Daniels, T. E., Mathis, K. J., Gobin, A. P., Lewis-de los Angeles, W. W., Smith, E. M., Chanthrakumar, P., de la Monte, S., & Tyrka, A. R. (2023). Associations of early life stress with leptin and ghrelin in healthy young adults. *Psychoneuroendocrinology, 149*, 106007. https://doi.org/10.1016/j.psyneuen.2022.106007

Darling Rasmussen, P., Storebø, O. J., Løkkeholt, T., Voss, L. G., Shmueli-Goetz, Y., Bojesen, A. B., Simonsen, E., & Bilenberg, N. (2019). Attachment as a core feature of resilience: A systematic review and meta-analysis. *Psychological Reports, 122*(4), 1259–1296. https://doi.org/10.1177/0033294118785577

de Lima, R. M., Barth, B., Mar Arcego, D., de Mendonça Filho, E. J., Patel, S., Wang, Z., Pokhvisneva, I., Parent, C., Levitan, R. D., Kobor, M. S., de Vasconcellos Bittencourt, A. P., Meaney, M. J., Dalmaz, C., & Silveira, P. P. (2022). Leptin receptor co-expression gene network moderates the effect of early life adversity on eating behavior in children. *Communications Biology, 5*(1). https://doi.org/10.1038/s42003-022-03992-8

Diener, E., Suh, E. M., Lucas, R. E., & Smith, H. L. (1999). Subjective Well-being: Three decades of progress. *Psychological Bulletin, 125*, 276–301. https://doi.org/10.1037/0033-2909.125.2.276

Dittus, P. J., Li, J., Verlenden, J. V., Wilkins, N. J., Carman-McClanahan, M. N., Cavalier, Y., Mercado, M. C., Welder, L. E., Roehler, D. R., & Ethier, K. A. (2023). Parental monitoring and risk Behaviors and experiences among high school students - youth risk behavior survey, United States, 2021. *MMWR Supplements, 72*(1), 37–44. https://doi.org/10.15585/mmwr.su7201a5

Felitti, V. J., Anda, R. F., Nordenberg, D., Williamson, D. F., Spitz, A. M., Edwards, V., Koss, M. P., & Marks, J. S. (1998). Relationship of childhood abuse and household dysfunction to many of the leading causes of death in adults. The adverse childhood experiences (ACE) study. *American Journal of Preventive Medicine, 14*(4), 245–258. https://doi.org/10.1016/s0749-3797(98)00017-8

Flaherty, S. C., & Sadler, L. S. (2011). A review of attachment theory in the context of adolescent parenting. *Journal of Pediatric Health Care, 25*(2), 114–121. https://doi.org/10.1016/j.pedhc.2010.02.005

Giano, Z., Wheeler, D. L., & Hubach, R. D. (2020). The frequencies and disparities of adverse childhood experiences in the U.S. *BMC Public Health, 20*(1), 1327. https://doi.org/10.1186/s12889-020-09411-z

Gundersen, C., & Ziliak, J. P. (2015). Food insecurity and health outcomes. *Health Affairs, 34*(11), 1830–1839. https://doi.org/10.1377/hlthaff.2015.0645

Hammons, A. J., & Fiese, B. H. (2011). Is frequency of shared family meals related to the nutritional health of children and adolescents? *Pediatrics, 127*(6), e1565–e1574. https://doi.org/10.1542/peds.2010-1440

Hantsoo, L., & Zemel, B. S. (2021). Stress gets into the belly: Early life stress and the gut microbiome. *Behavioural Brain Research, 414*, 113474. https://doi.org/10.1016/j.bbr.2021.113474

Harrist, A. W., Henry, C. S., Liu, C., & Morris, A. S. (2019). Family resilience: The power of rituals and routines in family adaptive systems. In B. Fiese, M. Celano, K. Deater-Deckard, E. N. Jouriles, & M. A. Whisman (Eds.), *The APA handbook of contemporary family psychology, volume 1: Foundations, methods, and changing forms* (pp. 223–239). American Psychological Association Press. https://doi.org/10.1037/0000099-013

Hasselle, A. J., Howell, K. H., Dormois, M., & Miller-Graff, L. E. (2017). The influence of childhood polyvictimization on disordered eating symptoms in emerging adulthood. *Child Abuse & Neglect, 68*, 55–64. https://doi.org/10.1016/j.chiabu.2017.04.003

Hays-Grudo, J., & Morris, A. S. (2020). *Adverse and protective childhood experiences: A developmental perspective*. American Psychological Association. https://doi.org/10.1037/0000177-000

Hays-Grudo, J., Morris, A. S., Beasley, L., Ciciolla, L., Shreffler, K., & Croff, J. (2021). Integrating and synthesizing adversity and resilience knowledge and action: The ICARE model. *American Psychologist, 76*(2), 203–215. https://doi.org/10.1037/amp0000766

Heckman, J. J. (2012). Invest in early childhood development: Reduce deficits, strengthen the economy. *The Heckman Equation, 7*(1–2).

Herman, J. P., McKlveen, J. M., Ghosal, S., Kopp, B., Wulsin, A., Makinson, R., Scheimann, J., & Myers, B. (2016). Regulation of the hypothalamic-pituitary-adrenocortical stress response. *Comprehensive Physiology, 6*(2), 603. https://doi.org/10.1002/cphy.c150015

Huang, J., & Barnidge, E. (2016). Low-income children's participation in the National School Lunch Program and household food insufficiency. *Social Science & Medicine, 150*, 8–14. https://doi.org/10.1016/j.socscimed.2015.12.020

Ibrahim Abdalla, M. M. (2015). Ghrelin - physiological functions and regulation. *European Endocrinology, 11*(2), 90–95. https://doi.org/10.17925/EE.2015.11.02.90

Jackson, D. B., Chilton, M., Johnson, K. R., & Vaughn, M. G. (2019). Adverse childhood experiences and household food insecurity: Findings from the 2016 National Survey of children's health. *American Journal of Preventive Medicine, 57*(5), 667–674. https://doi.org/10.1016/j.amepre.2019.06.004

John-Henderson, N. A., Henderson-Matthews, B., Ollinger, S. R., Racine, J., Gordon, M. R., Higgins, A. A., Horn, W. C., Reevis, S. A., Running Wolf, J. A., Grant, D., & Rynda-Apple, A. (2020). Adverse childhood experiences and immune system inflammation in adults residing on the Blackfeet reservation: The moderating role of sense of belonging to the community. *Annals of Behavioral Medicine, 54*(2), 87–93. https://doi.org/10.1093/abm/kaz029

Kazmierski, K. F. M., Borelli, J. L., & Rao, U. (2022). Negative affect, childhood adversity, and adolescents' eating following stress. *Appetite, 168*. https://doi.org/10.1016/j.appet.2021.105766

Knudsen, E. I. (2004). Sensitive periods in the development of the brain and behavior. *Journal of Cognitive Neuroscience, 16*(8), 1412–1425. https://doi.org/10.1162/0898929042304796

Luthar, S. S., Cicchetti, D., & Becker, B. (2000). The construct of resilience: A critical evaluation and guidelines for future work. *Child Development, 71*(3), 543–562. https://doi.org/10.1111/1467-8624.00164
Mahmood, L., Flores-Barrantes, P., Moreno, L. A., Manios, Y., & Gonzalez-Gil, E. M. (2021). The influence of parental dietary behaviors and practices on children's eating habits. *Nutrients, 13*(4), 1138. https://doi.org/10.3390/nu13041138
Mahoney, J. L., Cairns, B. D., & Farmer, T. W. (2003). Promoting interpersonal competence and educational success through extracurricular activity participation. *Journal of Educational Psychology, 95*, 409–418. https://doi.org/10.1037/0022-0663.95.2.409
Maniam, J., & Morris, M. J. (2010). Voluntary exercise and palatable high-fat diet both improve behavioural profile and stress responses in male rats exposed to early life stress: Role of hippocampus. *Psychoneuroendocrinology, 35*(10), 1553–1564. https://doi.org/10.1016/j.psyneuen.2010.05.012
Maslow, A. H. (1943). A theory of human motivation. *Psychological Review, 50*(4), 370–396. https://doi.org/10.1037/h0054346
Masten, A. S. (2001). Ordinary magic: Resilience processes in development. *American Psychologist, 56*(3), 227–238. 10.1037//0003-066X.56.3.227.
McEwen, B. S. (1998). Stress, adaptation, and disease. Allostasis and allostatic load. *Annals of the New York Academy of Sciences, 840*, 33–44. https://doi.org/10.1111/j.1749-6632.1998.tb09546.x
McLaughlin, K. A., & Hatzenbuehler, M. L. (2009). Stressful life events, anxiety sensitivity, and internalizing symptoms in adolescents. *Journal of Abnormal Psychology, 118*(3), 659. https://doi.org/10.1037/a0016499
McLaughlin, K. A., Koenen, K. C., Bromet, E. J., Karam, E. G., Liu, H., Petukhova, M., Meron Ruscio, A., Sampson, N. A., Stein, D. J., Aguilar-Gaxiola, S., Alonso, J., Borges, G., Demyttenaere, K., Dinolova, R. V., Ferry, F., Florescu, S., de Girolamo, G., Gureje, O., Kawakami, N., & Kessler, R. C. (2017). Childhood adversities and post-traumatic stress disorder: Evidence for stress sensitisation in the world mental health surveys. *The British Journal of Psychiatry, 211*(5), 280–288. https://doi.org/10.1192/bjp.bp.116.197640
Meaney, M. J. (2010). Epigenetics and the biological definition of gene × environment interactions. *Child Development, 81*(1), 41–79. https://doi.org/10.1111/j.1467-8624.2009.01381.x
Miller, G. E., Chen, E., & Parker, K. J. (2011). Psychological stress in childhood and susceptibility to the chronic diseases of aging: Moving toward a model of behavioral and biological mechanisms. *Psychological Bulletin, 137*(6), 959–997.
Miranda, M., Morici, J. F., Zanoni, M. B., & Bekinschtein, P. (2019). Brain-derived neurotrophic factor: A key molecule for memory in the healthy and the pathological brain. *Frontiers in Cellular Neuroscience, 13*, 363. https://doi.org/10.3389/fncel.2019.00363
Moon, I., & Han, J. (2022). Moderating effects of physical activity on the relationship between adverse childhood experiences and health-related quality of life. *International Journal of Environmental Research and Public Health, 19*(2), 668. https://doi.org/10.3390/ijerph19020668
Newman, B. M., Lohman, B. J., & Newman, P. R. (2007). Peer group membership and a sense of belonging: Their relationship to adolescent behavior problems. *Adolescence, 42*(166), 241–263.
Parade, S. H., Huffhines, L., Daniels, T. E., Stroud, L. R., Nugent, N. R., & Tyrka, A. R. (2021). A systematic review of childhood maltreatment and DNA methylation: Candidate gene and epigenome-wide approaches. *Translational Psychiatry, 11*(1), 134. https://doi.org/10.1038/s41398-021-01207-y
Petruccelli, K., Davis, J., & Berman, T. (2019). Adverse childhood experiences and associated health outcomes: A systematic review and meta-analysis. *Child Abuse & Neglect, 97*. https://doi.org/10.1016/j.chiabu.2019.104127
Pizzagalli, D. A. (2014). Depression, stress, and anhedonia: Toward a synthesis and integrated model. *Annual Review of Clinical Psychology, 10*, 393–423. https://doi.org/10.1146/annurev-clinpsy-050212-185606

Prior, A.-L., & Limbert, C. (2013). Adolescents' perceptions and experiences of family meals. *Journal of Child Health Care, 17*(4), 354–365. https://doi.org/10.1177/1367493512462261

Reid, B. M., Horne, R., Donzella, B., Szamosi, J. C., Coe, C. L., Foster, J. A., & Gunnar, M. R. (2021). Microbiota-immune alterations in adolescents following early life adversity: A proof of concept study. *Developmental Psychobiology, 63*(5), 851–863. https://doi.org/10.1002/dev.22061

Roth, T. L., & Sweatt, J. D. (2011). Epigenetic marking of the BDNF gene by early-life adverse experiences. *Hormones and Behavior, 59*(3), 315–320. https://doi.org/10.1016/j.yhbeh.2010.05.005

Satter, E. (1990). The feeding relationship: Problems and interventions. *The Journal of Pediatrics, 117*(2), S181–S189. https://doi.org/10.1016/S0022-3476(05)80017-4

Satter, E. M. (1995). Feeding dynamics: Helping children to eat well. *Journal of Pediatric Health Care, 9*, 178–184. https://doi.org/10.1016/s0891-5245(05)80033-1

Schore, A. N. (2001). Effects of a secure attachment relationship on right brain development, affect regulation, and infant mental health. *Infant Mental Health Journal, 22*(1–2), 7–66. https://doi.org/10.1002/1097-0355(200101/04)22:1<7::AID-IMHJ2>3.0.CO;2-N

Shankar, P., Chung, R., & Frank, D. (2017). Association of Food Insecurity with children's Behavioral, emotional, and academic outcomes: A systematic review. *Journal of Developmental & Behavioral Pediatrics, 38*(2), 135–150. https://doi.org/10.1097/DBP.0000000000000383

Simmons, B. L., Gooty, J., Nelson, D. L., & Little, L. M. (2009). Secure attachment: Implications for hope, trust, burnout, and performance. *Journal of Organizational Behavior, 30*(2), 233–247. https://doi.org/10.1002/job.585

Southwick, S. M., Morgan, C. A., III, Vythilingam, M., & Charney, D. (2007). Mentors enhance resilience in at-risk children and adolescents. *Psychoanalytic Inquiry, 26*(4), 577–584. https://doi.org/10.1080/07351690701310631

Spagnola, M., & Fiese, B. H. (2007). Family routines and rituals: A context for development in the lives of young children. *Infants & Young Children, 20*(4), 284–299. https://doi.org/10.1097/01.IYC.0000290352.32170.5a

Steinberg, D. B., & Simon, V. A. (2019). A comparison of hobbies and organized activities among low income urban adolescents. *Journal of Child and Family Studies, 28*, 1182–1195. https://doi.org/10.1007/s10826-019-01365-0

Stryzhak, O. O. (2020). The relationship between education, income, economic freedom and happiness. *SHS Web of Conferences, 75*. https://doi.org/10.1051/shsconf/20207503004

Suvarna, B., Suvarna, A., Phillips, R., Juster, R. P., McDermott, B., & Sarnyai, Z. (2020). Health risk behaviours and allostatic load: A systematic review. *Neuroscience and Biobehavioral Reviews, 108*, 694–711. https://doi.org/10.1016/j.neubiorev.2019.12.020

Teicher, M. H., Samson, J. A., Anderson, C. M., & Ohashi, K. (2016). The effects of childhood maltreatment on brain structure, function and connectivity. *Nature Reviews Neuroscience, 17*(10), 652. https://doi.org/10.1038/nrn.2016.111

United States Department of Agriculture. (2023). *Food insecurity and nutrition assistance*. https://www.ers.usda.gov/data-products/ag-and-food-statistics-charting-the-essentials/food-security-and-nutrition-assistance/#:~:text=In%202021%2C%2089.8%20percent%20of,had%20very%20low%20food%20security

Utter, J., Larson, N., Berge, J. M., Eisenberg, M. E., Fulkerson, J. A., & Neumark-Sztainer, D. (2018). Family meals among parents: Associations with nutritional, social and emotional wellbeing. *Preventive Medicine, 113*, 7–12. https://doi.org/10.1016/j.ypmed.2018.05.006

Van der Kolk, B. A. (2003). The neurobiology of childhood trauma and abuse. *Child and Adolescent Psychiatric Clinics, 12*(2), 293–317. https://doi.org/10.1016/S1056-4993(03)00003-8

Van Harmelen, A. L., Kievit, R. A., Ioannidis, K., Neufeld, S., Jones, P. B., Bullmore, E., Dolan, R., Fonay, P., Goodyer, I., & The NSPN Consortium. (2017). Adolescent friendships predict later resilient functioning across psychosocial domains in a healthy community cohort. *Psychological Medicine, 47*(13), 2312–2322. https://doi.org/10.1017/S0033291717000836

Vernon-Feagans, L., Willoughby, M., & Garrett-Peters, P. (2016). Predictors of behavioral regulation in kindergarten: Household chaos, parenting, and early executive functions. *Developmental Psychology, 52*(3), 430. https://doi.org/10.1037/dev0000087

Von Cheong, E., Sinnott, C., Dahly, D., & Kearney, P. M. (2017). Adverse childhood experiences (ACEs) and later-life depression: Perceived social support as a potential protective factor. *BMJ Open, 7*(9), e013228. https://doi.org/10.1136/bmjopen-2016-013228

Walsh, F. (2003). Family resilience: A framework for clinical practice. *Family Process, 42*(1), 1–18. https://doi.org/10.1111/j.1545-5300.2003.00001.x

Wren, A. M., & Bloom, S. R. (2007). Gut hormones and appetite control. *Gastroenterology, 132*(6), 2116–2130. https://doi.org/10.1053/j.gastro.2007.03.048

Yeung, J. W., Zhang, Z., & Kim, T. Y. (2018). Volunteering and health benefits in general adults: Cumulative effects and forms. *BMC Public Health, 18*(1), 1–8. https://doi.org/10.1186/s12889-017-4561-8

Yoon, C., Emery, R. L., Hazzard, V. M., Mason, S. M., & Neumark-Sztainer, D. (2022). Adverse experiences as predictors of maladaptive and adaptive eating: Findings from EAT 2018. *Appetite, 168*, 105737. https://doi.org/10.1016/j.appet.2021.105737

Chapter 2
The Role of Epigenetics and Early-Life Adversity in the Development of Obesity: Clinical and Animal Studies Perspective

Dolores Vazquez-Sanroman, Carolina Quijada, Olivia Zabel, and Jason Zabel

Approximately 20% of children in the United States are affected by obesity, yet practical solutions to combat this epidemic remain elusive (Brown et al., 2019) Prevention efforts over the past two decades have made minimal impact on curbing the rise of obesity among children (Mead et al., 2017). Traditional interventions focusing on energy balance and individual behavior changes, such as caloric restriction and increased physical activity, have not substantially reduced obesity rates. Prominent organizations like the National Collaborative for Childhood Obesity Research and the National Institutes of Health have advocated for a broader examination of social and environmental risk factors contributing to obesity (Brown et al., 2019).

Obesity has become a global health crisis, with its prevalence rising sharply in recent decades. Research on obesity emphasizes that genetics or environmental factors alone cannot fully explain their rise. Genetic studies have identified loci associated with body weight regulation, yet they fall short of describing the rapid increase in obesity. This gap suggests the critical role of environmental changes, such as diet, physical activity, and exposure to obesogenic chemicals (Baillie-Hamilton, 2002).

Research in the past four decades has described a possible link between the obesity epidemic and the proliferation of environmental factors, which can alter hormones, neurotransmitter sensitivity, and metabolic regulation, especially with early-life exposure. Moreover, the interplay between genetic predispositions and environmental exposures—gene–environment interactions—likely drives obesity trends, emphasizing the complexity of its etiology and the need for multidisciplinary research approaches to address this global challenge. While genetic studies have

D. Vazquez-Sanroman (✉) · C. Quijada · O. Zabel · J. Zabel
Department of Anatomy and Cell Biology, Oklahoma State University Center for Health Sciences, Tulsa, OK, USA
e-mail: dolores.vazquez_sanroman@okstate.edu

G. Welch et al. (eds.), *Stress, Resilience, and Healthy Relationships with Food and Family*, Emerging Issues in Family and Individual Resilience,
https://doi.org/10.1007/978-3-031-98937-7_2

identified numerous loci associated with body weight regulation, these findings cannot fully account for the dramatic increase in obesity rates, suggesting a significant role for environmental factors and gene–environmental interactions.

Research on environmental factors contributing to obesity highlights a vast and growing field. Key areas include the role of built environments, such as neighborhood access to nutritious foods and safe spaces for physical activity, and exposure to obesogens—chemicals that disrupt metabolic processes. Studies also emphasize the influence of food marketing, socioeconomic disparities, and urban design on obesity rates. Recent systematic reviews consolidate evidence showing these factors significantly impact individual and population-level weight outcomes, with new discoveries emerging yearly.

Adverse childhood experiences (ACEs), such as maltreatment or exposure to multiple stressors, are strongly correlated with obesity in later life. These early adversities disrupt the hypothalamus–pituitary–adrenal (HPA) axis, a critical regulator of the stress response, leading to epigenetic alterations in genes such as *NR3C1* and *FKBP5*. Such changes can impair cortisol regulation, promoting metabolic dysregulation, and lead to unhealthy coping behaviors like emotional eating. Concurrently, neurotrophic factors like BDNF, essential for neural plasticity and metabolic homeostasis, exhibit altered expression patterns in individuals with a history of ACEs, further linking early-life stress to obesity.

It is very important to highlight a gap in research. When attempting to define the relationship between ACEs, obesity, and epigenetics, there was a question as to the amount of research that has been dedicated to connecting the dots between all three components. Between 1999 and 2024, a large amount of research has explored the connection between ACEs and obesity, yielding 331 results on PubMed. Many papers have also been written relating ACEs to epigenetics, with 228 results seen on PubMed. Finally, an impressive amount of research has been done analyzing the relationship between obesity and epigenetics, with an astonishing 4830 results from PubMed. However, upon adding all three components to the PubMed search engine, only 13 papers are available, including 7 review articles. Thus, the primary objective of this chapter is to emphasize the necessity for high-quality primary research aimed at elucidating the potential relationship between ACEs, obesity, and epigenetic mechanisms. A clearer understanding of this connection could have significant clinical implications, contributing to a more comprehensive understanding of the long-term effects of ACEs and facilitating the development of more effective, targeted interventions for individuals globally.

Additionally, this review examines the interplay between epigenetic mechanisms and ACEs in the context of obesity, focusing on key pathways such as HPA axis dysregulation, neurotrophic signaling, and stress-related epigenetic modifications. By highlighting the molecular underpinnings of these relationships, we aim to provide insights into potential therapeutic strategies for addressing the complex intersection of ACEs, stress, and obesity.

2.1 Adverse Childhood Experiences

Adverse Childhood Experiences (ACEs) represent a potential risk factor for childhood obesity. ACEs are traumatic events occurring during childhood and are typically defined to include physical, psychological, or sexual abuse; neglect; exposure to family member substance abuse, mental illness, or criminal behavior; intimate partner violence against a female caregiver; and parental divorce, separation, or death (Felitti et al., 1998). Alarmingly, nearly half of children experience at least one ACE (Bethell et al., 2014; Horwitz, 1968; Snobl & Mydlil, 1973; Takayama et al., 1972). ACEs have been linked to a range of adverse health outcomes in adulthood, including cardiovascular disease and cancer. (Elsenburg et al., 2017; Hughes et al., 2017; Robson et al., 2020; Sramkiewicz & Prośba-Mackiewicz, 1987). Detrimental effects linked to ACEs often follow a dose–response pattern, with experiencing four or more ACEs correlating with a range of adverse health outcomes (Antoine & Lachapelle, 1988; Hughes et al., 2017; Jackson et al., 2022). However, their impact on childhood obesity is less well-studied than individual health behavior risk factors.

The relationship between ACEs and childhood obesity may involve multiple pathways through chronic or severe stress. ACEs can lead to neuroendocrine and physiological disruptions such as dysregulation of the hypothalamic–pituitary–adrenal (HPA) axis, altered hormonal responses to stress, and changes in appetite, with a preference for "comfort foods." Additionally, ACEs are associated with obesity-related behaviors, including poor impulse control, inadequate sleep, binge eating, and depression. Compounding stressors in the household and neighborhood environment can further obstruct a family's ability to promote healthy behaviors.

Several reviews have explored the link between ACEs and adult obesity, consistently finding an association. However, the connection between ACEs and childhood obesity is less understood, highlighting the need for further investigation. Given that nearly 50% of children experience ACEs and approximately 17% have obesity, a clearer understanding of the relationship between ACEs and childhood obesity is crucial. Research about the molecular mechanisms underlying ACEs has revealed that changes in epigenetic regulation such as DNA methylation may be related.

2.2 Epigenetic Changes

Epigenetics is an emerging area of biology that focuses on changes in gene expression that occur without alterations to the DNA sequence, instead involving chemical modifications of DNA and its associated proteins. These epigenetic mechanisms can have a profound impact on gene expression, cell differentiation, tissue development, and susceptibility to diseases. Gaining a deeper understanding of epigenetic changes is crucial for unraveling the mechanisms behind the increasing recognition of how environmental and lifestyle factors influence health, disease, and the inheritance of traits across generations. Recent research indicates that epigenetics plays a key role in various conditions, including cardiovascular disease, cancer, obesity, and neurodevelopmental and neurodegenerative disorders. Since epigenetic modifications are potentially reversible, they open up new possibilities for therapeutic treatments using epigenetic modulators.

Thus, epigenetics has emerged as a vital area of research in understanding how environmental exposures, particularly early-life adversity, influence obesity risk. If we understand that epigenetic mechanisms offer an additional layer of control over gene expression, allowing organisms to adapt to a changing environment, it is important to outline these alterations to examine their effects in the development and maintenance of obesity, especially if they contribute to treatment resistance or adherence. By modifying chromatin structure, nuclear organization, and transcript stability, epigenetic regulation enhances the functional complexity of DNA. These alterations can influence gene expression in ways that are either additive or synergistic, leading to long-lasting molecular and functional effects that are independent of the DNA sequence and may ultimately shape an organism's phenotype. The main epigenetic changes included: histone modification, DNA methylation, and the expression of small non-coding RNA species. In this chapter, we will describe histone modification and DNA methylation as are the epigenetic changes widely studied on relationship to obesity.

2.2.1 Histone Modification

Histone modification refers to the post-translational alteration of amino acid side chains in histone proteins. This process plays a key role in epigenetic regulation by influencing chromatin structure and modulating transcription factors' access to DNA, thereby affecting gene expression (Felsenfeld & Groudine, 2003). Human cells contain approximately 6.4 billion nucleotides distributed across 46 chromosomes (22 pairs of autosomes and two sex chromosomes). Due to its linear structure, DNA is far too long to fit within the confines of a cell nucleus without being compacted.

Chromatin, in a less compacted state, is organized into structural units called nucleosomes. Each nucleosome consists of eight histone proteins surrounded by a 150-nucleotide segment of DNA. The N-terminal regions of the histones, known as histone tails, extend outward from the nucleosome. These histone tails, made up of amino acids, undergo various post-translational modifications (Mersfelder & Parthun, 2006). These modifications influence essential cellular processes, including gene transcription, DNA repair, DNA replication, and chromatin condensation, by altering the chemical properties and physical structure of histones (Kouzarides, 2007). The impact of a specific histone modification depends on both the type of modification (e.g., acetylation, phosphorylation) and its location (e.g., the specific amino acid or position within the histone tail). These modifications can act independently, sequentially, or in combination, forming what is known as the "histone code." This code regulates access to specific DNA sequences, enabling distinct regulatory events (Zhang et al., 2021). A single modification can sometimes prevent other modifications from occurring at the same site. Additionally, histone modifications can influence protein binding to nearby amino acid side chains (Fischle et al., 2005) or affect an enzyme's ability to recognize neighboring sites (Clements et al., 2003).

2.2.2 *DNA Methylation*

DNA methylation involves the covalent attachment of a methyl group to a DNA nucleotide. This modification affects the ability of transcription factors and other DNA-binding proteins to recognize regulatory nucleotide sequences, often leading to the suppression of gene transcription (Hogg et al., 2020). Although DNA methylation is thought to occur across all organisms, the specific nucleotide and its position subject to methylation vary by species (Brown et al., 2019; Hattman, 2005). DNA methylation plays a critical role in normal development and cellular differentiation (Hattman, 2005). Although all nucleated cells in an organism share the same DNA sequence, methylation allows cells to differentiate and maintain their specific lineage by silencing or downregulating promoters of genes that are not required for a particular tissue. During cell division, DNA methylases help preserve the differentiated state by ensuring the methylation pattern is faithfully copied and passed on during mitosis.

In humans, DNA methylation occurs on cytosine nucleotides when they are immediately followed by guanine nucleotides in the 5′ direction. These cytosine–guanine sequences, linked by phosphate groups, are called CpG dinucleotides. On the complementary DNA strand, the CpG sequence is paired with a GpC sequence, and methylation is symmetrical, meaning that both cytosines in the pair are methylated (Ling & Rönn, 2019). CpG dinucleotides are often clustered in the promoter regions of many genes, forming what are known as CpG islands. These regions are defined as sequences with more than 50% guanine and cytosine content and a CpG-to-GpC ratio of at least 0.6 on the same strand (Deaton & Bird, 2011). The CpG dinucleotides that persist are often in regions where mutations would be harmful, such as gene promoters. For example, a mutation in a promoter's cytosine could disrupt transcription factor binding, alter gene expression, and affect the organism's phenotype and survival (Porcuna et al., 2021).

DNA methylation in gene promoters typically suppresses gene expression (Mahmoud, 2022). Conversely, active transcription occurs in the absence of methylation (Cuciureanu et al., 2023). Methylation represses gene expression through two primary mechanisms (Nishida et al., 2020). First, methylation in regulatory regions can block transcription factors from binding to DNA (Hark et al., 2000). Transcription factors, which bind specific DNA sequences in response to signals, recruit transcription machinery to enhance gene expression. When methylation occurs, this process is inhibited, preventing transcription initiation.

It is also possible that methylation in promoter regions increases the binding affinity of methyl-CpG-binding proteins, which outcompete transcription factors for binding to CpGs. These proteins physically block transcription factor access to the promoter, silencing the gene (Keller et al., 2020). Epigenetic control mechanisms may additively or synergistically interact to precisely respond to internal and external environmental cues. Determining the hierarchical relationships involved in epigenetic regulation and identifying mechanisms that are differentially expressed in different cell types will increase our understanding of gene expression and protein regulation.

2.3 Epigenetic Changes Associated with Obesity: What Do We Know?

The molecular mechanisms driving obesity have become of significant interest in biomedical and clinical research. This is especially relevant when we consider that obesity is a complex neurohormonal disorder stemming from disruptions in energy regulation pathways. It is associated with increased morbidity, mortality, and a diminished quality of life. The most prevalent form, polygenic obesity, arises from the interplay between multiple genetic variants and environmental factors. In contrast, monogenic and syndromic forms of obesity, which are caused by rare genetic mutations with limited environmental impact, can be distinguished by specific characteristics. Epigenetics changes in monogenic obesity compared to polygenic obesity are different.

Studies involving twins and families have highlighted the high heritability of obesity. At the same time, advances in mouse genetics have identified several essential genes linked to monogenic obesity, such as leptin (LEP), proopiomelanocortin (POMC), and melanocortin 4 receptor (MC4R) (van der Klaauw & Farooqi, 2015). These discoveries have enhanced our understanding of body weight regulation. However, for most individuals, obesity has a multigenetic and multifactorial epigenetic basis. Recent genome-wide association studies (GWAS) have identified numerous genes and single nucleotide polymorphisms (SNPs) associated with obesity (Loos & Yeo, 2022) though only a few have been reliably validated in follow-up studies. Importantly, genetics alone cannot account for the recent global rise in obesity rates. A tiny percentage of obese individuals carry mutations in the identified obesity-related genes, and it is improbable that the human genome has changed significantly in such a short time frame. Thus, it is evident that obesity arises from a complex interplay between genetic susceptibility and various environmental factors.

This has led to increasing interest in epigenetics, which helps bridge the gap between genes and environmental influences. Interestingly enough, recent reports also showed the role of FKBP5 (FKBP Prolyl Isomerase 5, a protein coding gene) methylation on responsiveness to exercise interventions (Willmer et al., 2022). Other genes, such as SCL6A3 (solute carrier family 6, neurotransmitter transporter, dopamine), member 3; in charge of dopamine transporter synthesis), SKA2 (spindle and kinetochore-associated protein 2, protein coding for cell proliferation and inflammation), and BDNF (brain derived-neurotrophic factor, pivotal for neuroplasticity and systemic inflammatory response), have also been implicated in stress mediation and obesity (Boks et al., 2016). Despite these findings, most studies have identified associations predominantly within specific demographic subgroups, leaving the underlying mechanisms largely unexplored (Miksza et al., 2023).

Epigenetics refers to heritable changes in gene expression that do not involve modifications to the DNA sequence itself. The term originated from Conrad Waddington's work aimed at explaining how cells with identical genomes can exhibit distinct specializations, such as hepatocytes and neurons, which differ significantly in their transcriptomic and proteomic profiles despite sharing the same DNA (Ruden et al., 2003). When epigenetics terminology is discussed, several mechanisms must be included, such as all post-translational modifications of histones and covalent modifications of DNA that shape chromatin structure (collectively referred to as epigenetic marks) (Table 2.1) (Erlich & Mills, 1985). In addition, non-coding RNAs have also been recognized as integral components of the epigenome (Nemeth et al., 2024). Through these mechanisms, cells can integrate environmental signals, coordinating a wide array of DNA processes, including gene

Table 2.1 Mechanisms of known epigenetic modifications in normal human development

Epigenetic modification	Enzymes involved	Genetic changes in function
CpG DNA methylation	DNA methyltransferases (DNMTs) 1, 3a, and 3b, along with base excision/DNA repair proteins or a failure to remethylate during DNA replication, are believed to contribute to demethylation	Their presence at promoters is linked to gene silencing, while their presence within gene bodies is associated with gene activity
Non-CpG DNA methylation	There is some evidence implicating well-established DNA methyltransferases	The exact role remains unclear, but its presence at genes is typically associated with gene activity
Histone acetylation	Multiple histone acetyltransferases (HATs) and histone deacetylases (HDACs)	Enhances protein access to DNA for transcription or genome-wide reprogramming
Histone methylation	Addition of methyl groups to lysine residues to activate or suppress transcription	Methylation of certain amino acid residues is associated with transcriptional repression, while others are linked to activation
Small non-coding RNAs, e.g. miRNAs, piRNA	The biogenesis and function of these molecules depend on enzymes like RNA polymerase II, DICER, and ARGONAUTE	A variety of effects, including transcriptional repression and activation, as well as translational repression

transcription pathways related to metabolic disease and enhanced our understanding of body weight regulation. However, for most individuals, obesity has a polygenic basis.

In 2014, Fall et al. performed one of the biggest genome-wide association studies in the European population with huge success in the identification of genetic loci affecting obesity and components of metabolic syndrome. Moreover, this study was a pioneer in the concept that common forms of obesity are highly polygenic, where numerous genes and single nucleotide polymorphisms (SNPs) associated with obesity can contribute to the development of metabolic syndrome (Liang et al., 2023). While epigenetic mechanisms are important, genetics alone cannot account for the recent global rise in obesity rates. A tiny percentage of obese individuals carry mutations in the identified obesity-related genes, and it is improbable that the human genome has changed significantly in such a short time frame. Thus, it is evident that obesity arises from a complex interplay between genetic susceptibility and various environmental factors. This has led to increasing interest in epigenetics, which helps bridge the gap between genes and environmental influences.

2.3.1 NR3C1: Glucocorticoids Role in Social Stress and Obesity

The stress sensitization theory suggests a connection between ACEs, later-life stress, and negative health outcomes. It posits that experiencing two or more ACEs disrupts the body's stress response systems, heightening sensitivity to future stressors. This early adversity can lead to exacerbated response to additional stressors, including additional adverse events, which may contribute to harmful health effects both immediately and later in life. The body's stress response is regulated by the hypothalamus–pituitary–adrenal (HPA) axis. This process begins with the hypothalamus releasing corticotropin-releasing factor (CRF), which stimulates the anterior pituitary to release adrenocorticotropic hormone (ACTH) into the bloodstream. ACTH, in turn, triggers the adrenal cortex to produce and release glucocorticoids (Epel et al., 2018).

The glucocorticoid receptor (GR or GCR) also known as NR3C1 (nuclear receptor subfamily 3, group C, member 1) gene encodes the glucocorticoid receptor (GR), which is crucial in regulating the HPA axis by interacting with cortisol and providing negative feedback to inhibit cortisol release (Berry et al., 2022). Methylation in the promoter region of this gene is linked to decreased GR expression and HPA dysregulation, which may contribute to the onset of psychiatric disorders in individuals facing psychosocial stress, early trauma, post-traumatic stress, gestational hunger, neglect, and other stressors. Furthermore, some researchers have suggested that NR3C1 methylation may also be associated with food intake, viewing it as a significant metabolic stress factor (Kiani et al., 2022). Obesity is a documented side effect of long-term glucocorticoid (GC) exposure, and GCs exert their physiological and pharmacological effect by binding to the nuclear receptor-glucocorticoid receptor (GR). A growing body of evidence suggests that GR responses to GCs function as a regulator for adipose metabolism, including adipogenesis and lipolysis (Meijer et al., 2018; Peckett et al., 2011; Shen et al., 2017). Elevated levels of cortisol in humans or corticosterone (CORT) in rodents suggest increased expression of NR3C1 and are associated with a CORT-induced obese phenotype (Porcuna et al., 2021).

The connection between epigenetic changes in the NR3C1 gene and ACEs is significant, particularly when considering obesity as a complex condition influenced by habits, behaviors, lifestyle, and overall health. Recent studies have shown a direct relationship between glucose levels, insulin resistance, and increased methylation patterns of the NR3C1 gene with age (de Souza et al., 2022). This suggests that lifestyle choices and life stressors can modulate the regulation of the NR3C1 gene through methylation, highlighting the intricate effects of the environment on stress reactivity (de Assis Pinheiro et al., 2021). Furthermore, chronic stress, linked to epigenetic alterations in NR3C1, can be induced by these factors changes (Borçoi et al., 2020). Mechanistically, a compelling hypothesis suggests that prolonged stress, such as that experienced from ACEs, disrupts the regulation of the HPA axis through negative feedback within the GR-cortisol complex, potentially leading to changes in stress reactivity and hypoactivation (Argentieri et al., 2017; Freitas et al., 2018). Lastly, a recent study demonstrated that increasing NR3C1 methylation levels correlated positively with a population that consumed a diet rich in highly processed food. Moreover, that specific group showed higher BMI, serum cortisol levels, and lipid profiles. Altogether, these results may indicate a relationship between NR3C1 methylation and metabolic changes related to the stress response.

2.3.2 BDNF, ACEs, and Obesity

As we discussed above, ACEs and obesity are interconnected, both influencing cognitive abilities like inhibitory control, mental flexibility, and working memory (Littleton et al., 2020). Despite that, the biological mechanisms linking higher levels of adversity and impaired cognition in obesity remain unclear. One potential factor for explaining the influence of ACEs in obesity is the neurotrophic factors, particularly brain-derived neurotrophic factor (BDNF). Along with nerve growth factor (NGF) and neurotrophins-3 and -4/5 (NT-3 and NT-4/5), brain-derived neurotrophic factor (BDNF) belongs to the neurotrophin family, which comprises small, secreted proteins crucial for vertebrate nervous system development, influencing cell proliferation, differentiation, survival, and essential behavioral functions. A defining characteristic of this family is a single coding exon, with complex expression due to multiple promoters and alternative splicing. BDNF is a neurotrophin essential for the development of plasticity in the central nervous system (CNS) (Lebrun et al., 2006). It is now recognized as a key player in regulating food intake. In addition to its crucial roles in neurological development, synaptic plasticity, learning, and memory, BDNF is vital for body weight regulation and energy homeostasis. Research has shown that individuals with obesity and type 2 diabetes often have low levels of circulating BDNF (Krabbe et al., 2007). Furthermore, there is an inverse relationship between peripheral BDNF concentrations and body mass index (BMI) in children and adults (Lommatzsch et al., 2005). Interestingly, in people with type 2 diabetes, plasma BDNF levels were lower regardless of obesity status, indicating that BDNF may influence obesity and insulin resistance through the modulation of leptin, insulin, and pancreatic polypeptide (PP) regulation (Pedersen et al., 2009).

BDNF isoforms, pro and mature BDNF, are biologically active, but their distinct roles are still being explored. BDNF has a well-documented association with mental health conditions, such as depression. Its serum levels and certain genetic variants (e.g., Val66Met polymorphism and T-allele carriers for variant rs10767664) have been linked to hippocampal size, memory recovery, and hypothalamic pathways that regulate body weight and responses to weight loss interventions (Egan et al., 2003). This suggests that BDNF plays a role in eating behaviors, body weight regulation, and insulin sensitivity.

Recently, our group demonstrated that higher ACEs-obesity index correlates with BDNF levels. Moreover, an important key outcome we found was that the relationship varied depending on whether we examined the mature form of BDNF or its precursor, proBDNF (Tavares & Tsotsoros, 2024). The mature BDNF is derived from proBDNF, and the two forms serve distinct biological functions. In our pilot sample, higher ACE scores were negatively associated with proBDNF levels. In contrast, mature BDNF levels were positively correlated with ACEs, suggesting a potential dose–response relationship for both forms. This pattern is consistent with findings from animal models of depression and chronic social defeat, where proBDNF expression was reduced and mature BDNF increased in brain regions associated with reward processing, such as the nucleus accumbens and amygdala. These divergent effects can be interpreted through the "yin-yang hypothesis," which posits that BDNF and proBDNF trigger opposing biological pathways. Specifically, proBDNF is associated with processes such as synaptic pruning, apoptosis, and long-term depression (LTD). In contrast, mature BDNF promotes the stabilization of neural terminals, activates the TrkB receptor, and plays a critical role in early long-term potentiation (LTP). Thus, our findings, if validated in more extensive studies, may suggest that individuals with higher levels of early-life adversity experience an increase in BDNF as an adaptive response to chronic stress. Given that BDNF expressions are essential for resilience to chronic stress and are modulated by corticosterone levels, these results could offer essential insights into the neurobiological mechanisms underpinning stress resilience.

The observed "see-saw" mechanism between proBDNF and mature BDNF may be better described as a bidirectional regulatory system in which the levels of each form of BDNF fluctuate in opposing directions, potentially balancing or counteracting each other's effects. This dynamic suggests a homeostatic feedback loop, where changes in one form of BDNF prompt compensatory changes in the other, helping the brain adapt to environmental factors such as stress or adversity. In this way, the system operates like a tug-of-war, with the two BDNF forms exerting opposing influences on neural processes to maintain functional stability. Our group and others have postulated a modest yet significant positive correlation between circulating proBDNF levels and neurocognitive performance. In individuals with obesity, reduced serum BDNF concentrations have been consistently associated with cognitive deficits, particularly in domains such as sustained attention, reaction time, and working memory. This association is especially pertinent given the integral role of fluid cognition and executive function in inhibitory control processes. Elevated proBDNF may contribute to enhanced cognitive function via its modulation of synaptic plasticity, dendritic remodeling, and long-term potentiation. Although mechanistic data elucidating this relationship remain limited, investigating neurobiological pathways that connect adverse childhood experiences (ACEs) with neural plasticity and cognitive outcomes in the context of obesity is critically important. The preliminary nature of current findings underscores the necessity for further empirical research to delineate the role of BDNF in the intersection of early-life stress and metabolic dysfunction.

2.3.3 FKBP5 Hypermethylation: A Missing Link

FK506-binding protein 5 (FKBP5) hypermethylation is an epigenetic mechanism linking ACEs to obesity and stress-related disorders. FKBP5, a key regulator of the stress response through its role in glucocorticoid receptor (GR) signaling, modulates the body's reaction to stress hormones like cortisol. Hypermethylation of FKBP5 CpG sites, often triggered by ACEs, reduces FKBP5 expression, impairing the feedback mechanism that normally regulates cortisol levels. This dysregulation leads to an elevated and prolonged stress response, contributing to physiological and behavioral changes such as altered reward processing and emotional eating, which increase the risk of obesity. While research highlights FKBP5's role in stress disorders, its methylation status in obesity and connection to ACEs remain underexplored. Understanding these links could inform targeted interventions addressing stress and metabolism.

There is growing evidence suggesting that early-life adversity, such as ACEs, can increase the risk of developing obesity later in life, partly through alterations in stress-related pathways. Individuals with hypermethylation of FKBP5 may be more vulnerable to the long-term effects of stress, which can manifest as unhealthy coping mechanisms. Studies in childhood trauma demonstrated that childhood physical abuse is associated with decreased methylation in one CpG of FKBP5 intron7 in offspring carrying the risk allele. Moreover, increased methylation of four FKBP5 CpG sites was associated with symptoms of depression, anxiety, and post-traumatic stress disorder (Yehuda et al., 2016). Interestingly, chronic activation of the hypothalamic–pituitary–adrenal (HPA) axis, resulting from dysregulated FKBP5 expression, can lead to higher levels of cortisol (Malekpour et al., 2023). Elevated cortisol, in turn, can promote fat storage, particularly in visceral fat depots, and interfere with appetite regulation, contributing to weight gain and obesity. Furthermore, the epigenetic modification of FKBP5 can have intergenerational effects (Bierer et al., 2020), meaning that ACEs experienced by one generation may lead to epigenetic changes in subsequent generations (Yehuda et al., 2016). This transgenerational inheritance of stress-related epigenetic marks, such as FKBP5 hypermethylation, may amplify the risk of obesity and related health outcomes across generations.

Understanding the role of FKBP5 hypermethylation in the relationship between ACEs and obesity has important implications for both prevention and treatment. If hypermethylation of FKBP5 contributes to the development of obesity, interventions aimed at modulating DNA methylation through lifestyle changes or pharmacological treatments targeting the stress response system could help mitigate the long-term health consequences of ACEs. Moreover, addressing the underlying psychosocial factors contributing to stress and trauma could prevent or reduce the impact of ACEs on the HPA axis and improve resilience against obesity.

2.3.4 Role of PPARγ

The need for further primary research pertaining to ACEs, obesity, and epigenetics is evident. In the limited primary literature sources described in Table 2.1, there were around 25 total biomarkers and genes potentially involved in the relationship between the above three components. Despite the limited data, epigenetic influence of PPARγ appears to have an underlying involvement with both ACEs and obesity among animal and human research studies. It is well-known that PPARγ plays a major role in adipose cell regulation and formation. Due to this role, it could provide a breakthrough for researchers to further investigate and find more data showing the influence that epigenetic modification of PPARγ has on the relationship between ACEs and obesity. Overall, the limited primary research on ACEs, obesity, and epigenetics has yielded promising results; yet, regarding PPARγ, pursuing future studies is necessary to be able to state with confidence that epigenetic modification of the gene plays a crucial role in bridging the gap between ACEs and obesity.

2.4 Conclusion

In conclusion, understanding the interplay between ACEs, obesity, and epigenetics is crucial for addressing the complex mechanisms underlying these interrelated phenomena. Although substantial research exists exploring the relationships between each pair of components, the integrated study of all three remains limited. This gap underscores the urgent need for comprehensive, high-quality primary research that bridges these domains.

The connection between ACEs and obesity involves multiple pathways, including neuroendocrine dysregulation, stress-induced behaviors, and epigenetic changes, such as methylation of key genes like NR3C1, BDNF, and FKBP5. These epigenetic modifications offer insights into how early-life adversity can shape long-term health outcomes, including metabolic dysregulation and altered stress reactivity. Meanwhile, obesity demonstrates a multifaceted etiology influenced by genetic predisposition, environmental factors, and epigenetic regulation. Together, these findings emphasize the intricate role of epigenetics as a mediator between environmental exposures and biological responses. This integrative approach has profound implications for clinical practice, public health interventions, and policymaking. By understanding how ACEs contribute to childhood and adult obesity through epigenetic mechanisms, researchers and clinicians can develop more targeted, effective interventions that address the root causes rather than just the symptoms of obesity. Moreover, such knowledge could inform prevention strategies aimed at mitigating the impact of ACEs on future generations, potentially breaking cycles of trauma and poor health. Ultimately, advancing the research on ACEs, obesity, and epigenetics could pave the way for novel therapeutic approaches, ranging from stress-regulation interventions to epigenetic-targeting treatments, fostering resilience and promoting better health outcomes across the lifespan.

Though current research remains limited with regard to the connection between ACEs, obesity, and epigenetics, there are still numerous implications for physicians to apply in any field of practice. In a primary care setting, doctors assess patients over a long period of time, thus permitting them to manage certain risk factors early on to prevent disease from setting in. For instance, a family medicine physician can discuss early interventions of obesity prevention, such as maintaining a balanced diet and exercise regimen, to a patient with multiple ACEs and epigenetic predispositions. In contrast, an orthopedic surgeon's familiarity with this subject will help him/her understand the possibility that a patient's early-life struggles may predispose him/her to obesity, which can have serious implications for various joints in the body. Learning that severe weight gain may not be simply due to food-driven impulses but rather could involve childhood trauma-induced DNA alterations will help individualize patient care and expand treatment options. Ultimately, the connection between ACEs, obesity, and epigenetics is complex and requires future studies; however, its understanding among physicians and other professionals will be vital in breaking down incorrect stereotypes that people struggling with obesity are simply making unhealthy habits.

Discussion Questions

1. How can an increased understanding of epigenetic changes in gene like NR3C1 and BDNF shape clinical practice to address childhood and adult obesity more effectively?
2. How can an increased understanding of epigenetic changes in gene like NR3C1 and BDNF shape public health policy to address childhood and adult obesity more effectively?

3. Considering the potential intergenerational impacts of epigenetic changes, how might this influence approaches to address obesity and ACEs in families and communities?
4. The chapter emphasizes the complexity of obesity's etiology, including epigenetic influences stemming from ACEs. How might this knowledge help reduce stigma and shift societal perceptions about obesity from one of individual responsibility to a more nuanced, systemic understanding?

References

Antoine, J. L., & Lachapelle, J. M. (1988). Variations in the quantities of petrolatum applied in patch testing. *Dermatosen in Beruf und Umwelt. Occupation and Environment, 36*(6), 191–194.

Argentieri, M. A., Nagarajan, S., Seddighzadeh, B., Baccarelli, A. A., & Shields, A. E. (2017). Epigenetic pathways in human disease: The impact of DNA methylation on stress-related pathogenesis and current challenges in biomarker development. *eBioMedicine, 18*, 327–350. https://doi.org/10.1016/j.ebiom.2017.03.044

Baillie-Hamilton, P. F. (2002). Chemical toxins: A hypothesis to explain the global obesity epidemic. *Journal of Alternative and Complementary Medicine, 8*(2), 185–192. https://doi.org/10.1089/107555302317371479

Berry, A., Mazzelli, M., Musillo, C., Riva, M. A., Cattaneo, A., & Cirulli, F. (2022). High-fat diet during adulthood interacts with prenatal stress, affecting both brain inflammatory and neuroendocrine markers in male rats. *The European Journal of Neuroscience, 55*(9–10), 2326–2340. https://doi.org/10.1111/ejn.15181

Bethell, C. D., Newacheck, P., Hawes, E., & Halfon, N. (2014). Adverse childhood experiences: Assessing the impact on health and school engagement and the mitigating role of resilience. *Health Affairs (Project Hope), 33*(12), 2106–2115. https://doi.org/10.1377/hlthaff.2014.0914

Bierer, L. M., Bader, H. N., Daskalakis, N. P., Lehrner, A., Provençal, N., Wiechmann, T., Klengel, T., Makotkine, I., Binder, E. B., & Yehuda, R. (2020). Intergenerational effects of maternal holocaust exposure on FKBP5 methylation. *The American Journal of Psychiatry, 177*(8), 744–753. https://doi.org/10.1176/appi.ajp.2019.19060618

Boks, M. P., Rutten, B. P. F., Geuze, E., Houtepen, L. C., Vermetten, E., Kaminsky, Z., & Vinkers, C. H. (2016). SKA2 methylation is involved in cortisol stress reactivity and predicts the development of post-traumatic stress disorder (PTSD) after military deployment. *Neuropsychopharmacology: Official Publication of the American College of Neuropsychopharmacology, 41*(5), 1350–1356. https://doi.org/10.1038/npp.2015.286

Borçoi, A. R., Mendes, S. O., Gasparini Dos Santos, J., Mota de Oliveira, M., Moreno, I. A. A., Freitas, F. V., Pinheiro, J. A., Arpini, J. K., Cunha, E. R., Archanjo, A. B., Monteiro, E., de Assis, A. L., Sorroche, B. P., Rebolho Batista Arantes, L. M., Borloti, E., & Álvares-da-Silva, A. M. (2020). Risk factors for depression in adults: NR3C1 DNA methylation and lifestyle association. *Journal of Psychiatric Research, 121*, 24–30. https://doi.org/10.1016/j.jpsychires.2019.10.011

Brown, T., Moore, T. H., Hooper, L., Gao, Y., Zayegh, A., Ijaz, S., Elwenspoek, M., Foxen, S. C., Magee, L., O'Malley, C., Waters, E., & Summerbell, C. D. (2019). Interventions for preventing obesity in children. *The Cochrane Database of Systematic Reviews, 7*(7), CD001871. https://doi.org/10.1002/14651858.CD001871.pub4

Clements, A., Poux, A. N., Lo, W.-S., Pillus, L., Berger, S. L., & Marmorstein, R. (2003). Structural basis for histone and phosphohistone binding by the GCN5 histone acetyltransferase. *Molecular Cell, 12*(2), 461–473. https://doi.org/10.1016/s1097-2765(03)00288-0

Cuciureanu, M., Carataşu, C.-C., Gabrielian, L., Frăsinariu, O. E., Checheriţă, L. E., Trandafir, L. M., Stanciu, G. D., Szilagyi, A., Pogonea, I., Bordeianu, G., Soroceanu, R. P., Andriţoiu, C. V., Anghel, M. M., Munteanu, D., Cernescu, I. T., & Tamba, B. I. (2023). 360-degree perspectives on obesity. *Medicina (Kaunas, Lithuania), 59*(6), 1119. https://doi.org/10.3390/medicina59061119

de Assis Pinheiro, J., Freitas, F. V., Borçoi, A. R., Mendes, S. O., Conti, C. L., Arpini, J. K., Dos Santos Vieira, T., de Souza, R. A., Dos Santos, D. P., Barbosa, W. M., Archanjo, A. B., de Oliveira, M. M., Dos Santos, J. G., Sorroche, B. P., Casali-da-Rocha, J. C., Trivilin, L. O., Borloti, E. B., Louro, I. D., Arantes, L. M. R. B., & Alvares-da-Silva, A. M. (2021). Alcohol consumption, depression, overweight and cortisol levels as determining factors for NR3C1 gene methylation. *Scientific Reports, 11*(1), 6768. https://doi.org/10.1038/s41598-021-86189-z

de Souza, M. L. M., Borçoi, A. R., Dutra, B. A. B., Dos Santos Vieira, T., Mendes, S. O., Moreno, I. A. A., Quaioto, B. R., Olinda, A. S., Cunha, E. R., Freitas, F. V., Pinheiro, J. A., Dos Santos, J. G., Sorroche, B. P., Arantes, L. M. R. B., Sartório, C. L., & da Silva, A. M. A. (2022). Lifestyle and NR3C1 exon 1F gene methylation is associated with changes in glucose levels and insulin resistance. *Life Sciences, 309*, 120940. https://doi.org/10.1016/j.lfs.2022.120940

Deaton, A. M., & Bird, A. (2011). CpG islands and the regulation of transcription. *Genes & Development, 25*(10), 1010–1022. https://doi.org/10.1101/gad.2037511

Egan, M. F., Kojima, M., Callicott, J. H., Goldberg, T. E., Kolachana, B. S., Bertolino, A., Zaitsev, E., Gold, B., Goldman, D., Dean, M., Lu, B., & Weinberger, D. R. (2003). The BDNF val66met polymorphism affects activity-dependent secretion of BDNF and human memory and hippocampal function. *Cell, 112*(2), 257–269. https://doi.org/10.1016/s0092-8674(03)00035-7

Elsenburg, L. K., van Wijk, K. J. E., Liefbroer, A. C., & Smidt, N. (2017). Accumulation of adverse childhood events and overweight in children: A systematic review and meta-analysis. *Obesity Reviews, 18*(11), 1325–1335. https://doi.org/10.1111/obr.12555

Epel, E. S., Crosswell, A. D., Mayer, S. E., Prather, A. A., Slavich, G. M., Puterman, E., & Mendes, W. B. (2018). More than a feeling: A unified view of stress measurement for population science. *Frontiers in Neuroendocrinology, 49*, 146–169. https://doi.org/10.1016/j.yfrne.2018.03.001

Erlich, K. S., & Mills, J. (1985). Chemotherapy for herpes simplex virus infections. *The Western Journal of Medicine, 143*(5), 648–655.

Felitti, V. J., Anda, R. F., Nordenberg, D., Williamson, D. F., Spitz, A. M., Edwards, V., Koss, M. P., & Marks, J. S. (1998). Relationship of childhood abuse and household dysfunction to many of the leading causes of death in adults. The adverse childhood experiences (ACE) study. *American Journal of Preventive Medicine, 14*(4), 245–258. https://doi.org/10.1016/s0749-3797(98)00017-8

Felsenfeld, G., & Groudine, M. (2003). Controlling the double helix. *Nature, 421*(6921), 448–453. https://doi.org/10.1038/nature01411

Fischle, W., Tseng, B. S., Dormann, H. L., Ueberheide, B. M., Garcia, B. A., Shabanowitz, J., Hunt, D. F., Funabiki, H., & Allis, C. D. (2005). Regulation of HP1-chromatin binding by histone H3 methylation and phosphorylation. *Nature, 438*(7071), 1116–1122. https://doi.org/10.1038/nature04219

Freitas, F. V., Barbosa, W. M., Silva, L. A. A., de Garozi, M. J. O., de Pinheiro, J. A., Borçoi, A. R., Conti, C. L., Arpini, J. K., de Paula, H., de Oliveira, M. M., Archanjo, A. B., de Freitas, É. A. S., de Oliveira, D. R., Borloti, E. B., Louro, I. D., & Alvares-da-Silva, A. M. (2018). Psychosocial stress and central adiposity: A Brazilian study with a representative sample of the public health system users. *PLoS One, 13*(7), e0197699. https://doi.org/10.1371/journal.pone.0197699

Hark, A. T., Schoenherr, C. J., Katz, D. J., Ingram, R. S., Levorse, J. M., & Tilghman, S. M. (2000). CTCF mediates methylation-sensitive enhancer-blocking activity at the H19/Igf2 locus. *Nature, 405*(6785), 486–489. https://doi.org/10.1038/35013106

Hattman, S. (2005). DNA-[adenine] methylation in lower eukaryotes. *Biochemistry. Biokhimiia, 70*(5), 550–558. https://doi.org/10.1007/s10541-005-0148-6

Hogg, S. J., Beavis, P. A., Dawson, M. A., & Johnstone, R. W. (2020). Targeting the epigenetic regulation of antitumour immunity. *Nature Reviews. Drug Discovery, 19*(11), 776–800. https://doi.org/10.1038/s41573-020-0077-5

Horwitz, A. (1968). Education of health specialists in the Americas. *Boletin De La Oficina Sanitaria Panamericana. Pan American Sanitary Bureau, 64*(2), 154–156.

Hughes, K., Bellis, M. A., Hardcastle, K. A., Sethi, D., Butchart, A., Mikton, C., Jones, L., & Dunne, M. P. (2017). The effect of multiple adverse childhood experiences on health: A systematic review and meta-analysis. *The Lancet. Public Health, 2*(8), e356–e366. https://doi.org/10.1016/S2468-2667(17)30118-4

Jackson, D. B., Testa, A., Woodward, K. P., Qureshi, F., Ganson, K. T., & Nagata, J. M. (2022). Adverse childhood experiences and cardiovascular risk among young adults: Findings from the 2019 Behavioral risk factor surveillance system. *International Journal of Environmental Research and Public Health, 19*(18), 11710. https://doi.org/10.3390/ijerph191811710

Keller, M., Yaskolka Meir, A., Bernhart, S. H., Gepner, Y., Shelef, I., Schwarzfuchs, D., Tsaban, G., Zelicha, H., Hopp, L., Müller, L., Rohde, K., Böttcher, Y., Stadler, P. F., Stumvoll, M., Blüher, M., Kovacs, P., & Shai, I. (2020). DNA methylation signature in blood mirrors successful weight-loss during lifestyle interventions: The CENTRAL trial. *Genome Medicine, 12*(1), 97. https://doi.org/10.1186/s13073-020-00794-7

Kiani, A. K., Bonetti, G., Donato, K., Kaftalli, J., Herbst, K. L., Stuppia, L., Fioretti, F., Nodari, S., Perrone, M., Chiurazzi, P., Bellinato, F., Gisondi, P., & Bertelli, M. (2022). Polymorphisms, diet and nutrigenomics. *Journal of Preventive Medicine and Hygiene, 63*(2 Suppl 3), E125–E141. https://doi.org/10.15167/2421-4248/jpmh2022.63.2S3.2754

Kouzarides, T. (2007). Chromatin modifications and their function. *Cell, 128*(4), 693–705. https://doi.org/10.1016/j.cell.2007.02.005

Krabbe, K. S., Nielsen, A. R., Krogh-Madsen, R., Plomgaard, P., Rasmussen, P., Erikstrup, C., Fischer, C. P., Lindegaard, B., Petersen, A. M. W., Taudorf, S., Secher, N. H., Pilegaard, H., Bruunsgaard, H., & Pedersen, B. K. (2007). Brain-derived neurotrophic factor (BDNF) and type 2 diabetes. *Diabetologia, 50*(2), 431–438. https://doi.org/10.1007/s00125-006-0537-4

Lebrun, B., Bariohay, B., Moyse, E., & Jean, A. (2006). Brain-derived neurotrophic factor (BDNF) and food intake regulation: A minireview. *Autonomic Neuroscience: Basic & Clinical, 126–127*, 30–38. https://doi.org/10.1016/j.autneu.2006.02.027

Liang, Y. Y., Chen, J., Peng, M., Zhou, J., Chen, X., Tan, X., Wang, N., Ma, H., Guo, L., Zhang, J., Wing, Y.-K., Geng, Q., & Ai, S. (2023). Association between sleep duration and metabolic syndrome: Linear and nonlinear Mendelian randomization analyses. *Journal of Translational Medicine, 21*(1), 90. https://doi.org/10.1186/s12967-023-03920-2

Ling, C., & Rönn, T. (2019). Epigenetics in human obesity and type 2 diabetes. *Cell Metabolism, 29*(5), 1028–1044. https://doi.org/10.1016/j.cmet.2019.03.009

Littleton, S. H., Berkowitz, R. I., & Grant, S. F. A. (2020). Genetic determinants of childhood obesity. *Molecular Diagnosis & Therapy, 24*(6), 653–663. https://doi.org/10.1007/s40291-020-00496-1

Lommatzsch, M., Zingler, D., Schuhbaeck, K., Schloetcke, K., Zingler, C., Schuff-Werner, P., & Virchow, J. C. (2005). The impact of age, weight and gender on BDNF levels in human platelets and plasma. *Neurobiology of Aging, 26*(1), 115–123. https://doi.org/10.1016/j.neurobiolaging.2004.03.002

Loos, R. J. F., & Yeo, G. S. H. (2022). The genetics of obesity: From discovery to biology. *Nature Reviews. Genetics, 23*(2), 120–133. https://doi.org/10.1038/s41576-021-00414-z

Mahmoud, A. M. (2022). An overview of epigenetics in obesity: The role of lifestyle and therapeutic interventions. *International Journal of Molecular Sciences, 23*(3), 1341. https://doi.org/10.3390/ijms23031341

Malekpour, M., Shekouh, D., Safavinia, M. E., Shiralipour, S., Jalouli, M., Mortezanejad, S., Azarpira, N., & Ebrahimi, N. D. (2023). Role of FKBP5 and its genetic mutations in stress-induced psychiatric disorders: An opportunity for drug discovery. *Frontiers in Psychiatry, 14*, 1182345. https://doi.org/10.3389/fpsyt.2023.1182345

Mead, E., Brown, T., Rees, K., Azevedo, L. B., Whittaker, V., Jones, D., Olajide, J., Mainardi, G. M., Corpeleijn, E., O'Malley, C., Beardsmore, E., Al-Khudairy, L., Baur, L., Metzendorf, M.-I., Demaio, A., & Ells, L. J. (2017). Diet, physical activity and behavioural interventions for the treatment of overweight or obese children from the age of 6 to 11 years. *The Cochrane Database of Systematic Reviews, 6*(6), CD012651. https://doi.org/10.1002/14651858.CD012651

Meijer, O. C., Koorneef, L. L., & Kroon, J. (2018). Glucocorticoid receptor modulators. *Annales D'endocrinologie, 79*(3), 107–111. https://doi.org/10.1016/j.ando.2018.03.004

Mersfelder, E. L., & Parthun, M. R. (2006). The tale beyond the tail: Histone core domain modifications and the regulation of chromatin structure. *Nucleic Acids Research, 34*(9), 2653–2662. https://doi.org/10.1093/nar/gkl338

Miksza, U., Adamska-Patruno, E., Bauer, W., Fiedorczuk, J., Czajkowski, P., Moroz, M., Drygalski, K., Ustymowicz, A., Tomkiewicz, E., Gorska, M., & Kretowski, A. (2023). Obesity-related parameters in carriers of some BDNF genetic variants may depend on daily dietary macronutrients intake. *Scientific Reports, 13*(1), 6585. https://doi.org/10.1038/s41598-023-33842-4

Nemeth, K., Bayraktar, R., Ferracin, M., & Calin, G. A. (2024). Non-coding RNAs in disease: From mechanisms to therapeutics. *Nature Reviews. Genetics, 25*(3), 211–232. https://doi.org/10.1038/s41576-023-00662-1

Nishida, H., Onishi, K., Kurose, S., Tsutsumi, H., Miyauchi, T., Takao, N., Yoshiuchi, S., Fujii, A., & Kimura, Y. (2020). Changes in body composition and FTO whole blood DNA methylation among Japanese women: A randomized clinical trial of weight-loss program. *Diabetes, Metabolic Syndrome and Obesity: Targets and Therapy, 13*, 2157–2167. https://doi.org/10.2147/DMSO.S248769

Peckett, A. J., Wright, D. C., & Riddell, M. C. (2011). The effects of glucocorticoids on adipose tissue lipid metabolism. *Metabolism: Clinical and Experimental, 60*(11), 1500–1510. https://doi.org/10.1016/j.metabol.2011.06.012

Pedersen, B. K., Pedersen, M., Krabbe, K. S., Bruunsgaard, H., Matthews, V. B., & Febbraio, M. A. (2009). Role of exercise-induced brain-derived neurotrophic factor production in the regulation of energy homeostasis in mammals. *Experimental Physiology, 94*(12), 1153–1160. https://doi.org/10.1113/expphysiol.2009.048561

Porcuna, J., Mínguez-Martínez, J., & Ricote, M. (2021). The PPARα and PPARγ epigenetic landscape in cancer and immune and metabolic disorders. *International Journal of Molecular Sciences, 22*(19), 10573. https://doi.org/10.3390/ijms221910573

Robson, D. A., Allen, M. S., & Howard, S. J. (2020). Self-regulation in childhood as a predictor of future outcomes: A meta-analytic review. *Psychological Bulletin, 146*(4), 324–354. https://doi.org/10.1037/bul0000227

Ruden, D. M., Garfinkel, M. D., Sollars, V. E., & Lu, X. (2003). Waddington's widget: Hsp90 and the inheritance of acquired characters. *Seminars in Cell & Developmental Biology, 14*(5), 301–310. https://doi.org/10.1016/j.semcdb.2003.09.024

Shen, Y., Roh, H. C., Kumari, M., & Rosen, E. D. (2017). Adipocyte glucocorticoid receptor is important in lipolysis and insulin resistance due to exogenous steroids, but not insulin resistance caused by high fat feeding. *Molecular Metabolism, 6*(10), 1150–1160. https://doi.org/10.1016/j.molmet.2017.06.013

Snobl, O., & Mydlil, V. (1973). Problems of diagnosis of megacolon in neonatal period (functional pseudomegacolon in a premature infant). *Ceskoslovenska Pediatrie, 28*(4), 197–200.

Sramkiewicz, J., & Prośba-Mackiewicz, M. (1987). Prosthetic treatment of patients with soft palate defects. *Protetyka Stomatologiczna, 37*(3), 115–121.

Takayama, K., Wang, L., & David, H. L. (1972). Effect of isoniazid on the in vivo mycolic acid synthesis, cell growth, and viability of mycobacterium tuberculosis. *Antimicrobial Agents and Chemotherapy, 2*(1), 29–35. https://doi.org/10.1128/AAC.2.1.29

Tavares, K. L., & Tsotsoros, C. E. (2024). The relation between adverse childhood experiences and health behaviors in adult women. *American Journal of Health Promotion: AJHP, 38*(6), 778–786. https://doi.org/10.1177/08901171241229829

van der Klaauw, A. A., & Farooqi, I. S. (2015). The hunger genes: Pathways to obesity. *Cell, 161*(1), 119–132. https://doi.org/10.1016/j.cell.2015.03.008

Willmer, T., Oosthuizen, A., Dias, S., Mendham, A. E., Goedecke, J. H., & Pheiffer, C. (2022). A pilot investigation of genetic and epigenetic variation of FKBP5 and response to exercise intervention in African women with obesity. *Scientific Reports, 12*(1), 11771. https://doi.org/10.1038/s41598-022-15678-6

Yehuda, R., Daskalakis, N. P., Bierer, L. M., Bader, H. N., Klengel, T., Holsboer, F., & Binder, E. B. (2016). Holocaust exposure induced intergenerational effects on FKBP5 methylation. *Biological Psychiatry, 80*(5), 372–380. https://doi.org/10.1016/j.biopsych.2015.08.005

Zhang, Y., Sun, Z., Jia, J., Du, T., Zhang, N., Tang, Y., Fang, Y., & Fang, D. (2021). Overview of histone modification. *Advances in Experimental Medicine and Biology, 1283*, 1–16. https://doi.org/10.1007/978-981-15-8104-5_1

Chapter 3
Parents' Information Seeking and Use Regarding Infant and Toddler Nutrition Topics: A Conceptual Model and Empirical Example of Information Behavior

Allison Doub Hepworth, Meg L. Small, and Timothy R. Brick

Adequate nutrition is essential for human well-being throughout the lifespan and is especially important during the first 2 years of life, which is a time of rapid physical and cognitive growth (Birch & Doub, 2014). For many parents and other primary caregivers in the United States (U.S.), the arrival of their first child marks the first time that they are entirely responsible for infant care and feeding. Fewer natural opportunities exist in the U.S. to participate in and observe infant care compared to many non-Western countries (Hadley et al., 2010; Reupert et al., 2022). Therefore, first-time parents often develop and refine their knowledge, beliefs, and behaviors related to child feeding as their child develops. While many factors influence child feeding, parents' information behavior contributes to the knowledge, skills, and resources that determine what and how they feed their children.

Information behavior is a comprehensive term that encompasses all human interactions with information, including information needs, intentional information seeking, serendipitous information exposure, information avoidance, information processing, information use, and information evaluation (Given et al., 2023, pp. 1–18). For example, a parent notices that their 2-year-old child is rejecting vegetables, which creates an information need for advice about increasing toddler vegetable intake. The parent intentionally seeks information by searching websites and

A. D. Hepworth (✉)
Department of Nutritional Sciences, Oklahoma State University, Stillwater, OK, USA
e-mail: allison.hepworth@okstate.edu

M. L. Small
College of Health and Human Development, Pennsylvania State University, University Park, PA, USA

T. R. Brick
Department of Human Development and Family Studies, Pennsylvania State University, University Park, PA, USA

G. Welch et al. (eds.), *Stress, Resilience, and Healthy Relationships with Food and Family*, Emerging Issues in Family and Individual Resilience,
https://doi.org/10.1007/978-3-031-98937-7_3

social media for advice. During this search, the parent finds a blog post on ways to incorporate blended vegetables into recipes such as smoothies and muffins. The parent processes the information and decides to blend vegetables into a smoothie using a recipe they found. The toddler enjoys the smoothie, and the parent views it as a success in increasing vegetable intake. The parent may continue searching for more recipes to add variety.

The nutrition knowledge that parents gain and apply during infancy and toddlerhood has lasting effects on child health. For example, maternal diet during pregnancy and breastfeeding influences birthweight, neurological development, and flavor acceptance (Marshall et al., 2022), and longer breastfeeding duration reduces risks of infections and childhood obesity (Pattison et al., 2019). Bottle feeding practices, such as formula choice and feeding frequency, and the timing of introducing solid foods, including potential allergens, influence growth patterns and allergy risks (D'Hollander et al., 2022; Scarpone et al., 2023; Totzauer et al., 2022; Ventura & Whaley, 2022). Additionally, food parenting practices, such as pressuring, restricting, or being responsive to child eating cues, affect a child's ability to self-regulate eating (Spill et al., 2019). Parenting behaviors related to sleep, physical activity, and screen time, which are linked to feeding, also impact growth and eating habits (Brown & Harries, 2015; Carson et al., 2017; Janssen et al., 2020). The long-term effects of nutrition during infancy and early childhood demonstrate the relevance of parents' information behavior to family resilience.

Family resilience broadly refers to a family's ability to successfully navigate life's challenges (Masten, 2018; Patterson, 2002). Families are interdependent systems in which each family member influences and is influenced by the other members. The family system is embedded within broader social systems, such as local communities and political environments, that impact collective well-being. Family resilience includes the strengths and resources that family members can leverage to prevent or respond to situations that threaten well-being (Henry et al., 2015). The ability of parents to access, interpret, and apply accurate nutrition and health information can build family resilience by empowering parents to make informed decisions and connect them to resources that help to maintain or improve the family's well-being. Identifying factors that support information behaviors that promote the uptake of evidence-based information regarding infant nutrition could strengthen family resilience.

3.1 Literature Review

This literature review presents the current nutrition recommendations for infants and toddlers as of August 2024, covering topics such as breastfeeding, introducing complementary and allergenic foods, and dietary patterns for toddlers aged 12–23 months. It also explores the connection between parents' information-seeking behaviors and their infant and toddler feeding practices. A new conceptual model of information behavior is introduced, offering testable predictions on how individuals seek, process, and use information, shaped by their needs, motivations, abilities, and surrounding socioecological context and information environment. Examples of the model's application to infant and toddler feeding are highlighted throughout.

3.1.1 Infant and Toddler Feeding Recommendations

The ninth edition of the *Dietary Guidelines for Americans, 2020–2025* were the first to include nutrition recommendations for infants and toddlers from birth to 24 months (U.S. Department of Agriculture (USDA) and U.S. Department of Health and Human Services (HHS), 2020). The American Academy of Pediatrics also disseminates evidence-based nutrition guidance through pediatric healthcare professionals and directly to parents, for example, through their policy statement, *Breastfeeding and the Use of Human Milk* (Meek et al., 2022). While the *Dietary Guidelines for Americans, 2020–2025* and the American Academy of Pediatrics specify health-promoting feeding practices for infants and toddlers, recommendations for what and how to feed children under age 2 years are still limited by a lack of evidence from controlled trials (Zimmer et al., 2023). As described in detail in the cited articles that follow each topic, more evidence is especially needed on factors that influence human breastmilk production and composition (Donovan et al., 2023), how infant formula compositions influence child growth and metabolism (Lemaire et al., 2018), how the timing and order of solid food introduction influences later food acceptance and diet quality (Johnson et al., 2022; Moding & Kielb, 2023), and what specific feeding practices promote children's eating competence and diet quality (Balantekin et al., 2020; Langdon-Daly & Serpell, 2017). As evidence on these and other topics accrues, guidance on infant and toddler nutrition will continue to evolve accordingly.

The evolving information landscape on infant and toddler nutrition requires parents, caregivers, and healthcare professionals to stay current on the most recent recommendations. Otherwise, outdated feeding practices could continue which negatively affect children's mental and/or physical well-being. For example, chronically pressuring children to eat all of the food served to them (i.e., "clean your plate") is a controlling and intrusive feeding practice that likely evolved to protect children from undernutrition and food scarcity but is now considered a risk factor for eating dysregulation (Ellis et al., 2016; Savage et al., 2007). Instead, the *Dietary Guidelines for Americans, 2020–2025* advises parents to use responsive feeding practices that support children's abilities to notice and respond to their internal hunger and fullness cues (Black & Aboud, 2011; USDA and HHS, 2020). Recommendations for breastfeeding duration and introducing complementary foods (i.e., any foods and beverages other than breastmilk or infant formula), including potentially allergenic foods, and dietary patterns for children ages 12–23 months have also been recently updated and are described below.

3.1.2 Breastfeeding Recommendations

Breastmilk provides optimal nutrition for infants and is associated with numerous maternal and child health benefits throughout the lifespan (Meek et al., 2022). The American Academy of Pediatrics recommends exclusively breastfeeding for 6 months, with continued breastfeeding for 2 years or longer if mutually desired (Meek et al., 2022). The most recent statistics reported in the Centers for Disease Control and Prevention (CDC) *Breastfeeding Report Card United States, 2022* indicated that among infants born in 2019, the majority of infants (83%) were breastfed at birth, but only about one-in-four infants were exclusively breastfed at age 6 months, and only about one-in-three received any breastmilk at age 12 months (CDC, 2022). Estimates for breastfeeding at age 24 months should be in future reports to reflect the updated guidance.

3.1.3 Introducing Complementary Foods Recommendations

The *Dietary Guidelines for Americans, 2020–2025* recommend introducing complementary foods around age 6 months, and not before age 4 months, depending on signs of developmental readiness (USDA and HHS, 2020). Data from the National Health and Nutrition Examination Survey (2016–2018) showed that approximately two-thirds of parents introduced complementary foods between ages 4 and 6 months, with approximately one-third introducing complementary foods during the sixth month of life (Chiang et al., 2023). Approximately 15% of parents introduced complementary foods before age 4 months and approximately 21% introduced complementary foods after age 7 months (Chiang et al., 2023). Early introduction of solid foods can negatively impact the child's developing digestive tract and has been correlated with higher childhood obesity risk in some studies, although more research is needed to clarify how, when, and what solid foods introduced impact infant growth (D'Hollander et al., 2022; Daniels et al., 2015). Introducing solid foods later than recommended can lead to increasing the child's difficulty in accepting different food textures, especially if introduced after age 9 months (Johnson et al., 2018).

3.1.4 Introducing Potentially Allergenic Foods Recommendations

The *Dietary Guidelines for Americans, 2020–2025* recommend introducing potentially allergenic foods along with other complementary foods around age 6 months in developmentally appropriate forms (USDA and HHS, 2020). Children at high risk for peanut allergy, as indicated by severe eczema, egg allergy, or both, should be introduced to age-appropriate peanut-containing foods between ages 4 and

6 months in consultation with their child's healthcare provider (USDA and HHS, 2020). The mechanisms that explain why earlier introduction to potentially allergenic food decreases the risk of developing allergies are still being investigated (Krawiec et al., 2021). A survey conducted in 2021 showed that by age 7 months, only 50% of U.S. parents had introduced ≥1 potentially allergenic food, and less than 1% had introduced all top nine food allergens (Venter et al., 2022). By age 13 months, 94% of parents had introduced ≥1 of the top nine food allergens, but only 2.5% had introduced all nine (Venter et al., 2022). These data show that many caregivers need more information and support in offering potentially allergenic foods.

The nine most common food allergens are cow's milk, eggs, peanuts, tree nuts (almonds, Brazil nuts, cashews, hazelnuts, pecans, pistachios, and walnuts), fish, crustacean shellfish, wheat, soy, and sesame (U.S. Food & Drug Administration, 2023). Whole peanuts and peanut butter are choking hazards to children under age 4 years, so caregivers must introduce peanuts in developmentally appropriate ways. One recommended option is to mix 2 teaspoons of smooth (not chunky) peanut butter with 2–3 teaspoons of hot water and to allow the mixture to cool prior to offering a small taste to the infant (Togias et al., 2017). If there are no signs of an allergic response within 10 minutes (e.g., vomiting, hives, difficulty breathing), the infant can continue to eat the rest of the food (Togias et al., 2017). Infants who are tolerating potentially allergenic foods should be offered them on a regular basis (e.g., a few times a week), although there are no precise recommendations for how frequently they should be offered (USDA and HHS, 2020).

3.1.5 Dietary Pattern Recommendations

The *Dietary Guidelines for Americans, 2020–2025* were the first to recommend specific dietary patterns for toddlers ages 12–23 months (USDA and HHS, 2020). There are no specific dietary pattern recommendations for infants ages 6 to 11 months because of limited evidence and wide variations in infant consumption of breastmilk and/or infant formula as parents introduce complementary foods (USDA and HHS, 2020; Zimmer et al., 2023). For children ages 12–23 months, the general recommendations are to offer toddlers a variety of nutrient-dense foods from each food group (i.e., protein foods, dairy, vegetables, fruits, grains), avoid offering any foods or beverages with added sugars before age 2 years, and avoid offering foods higher in sodium (USDA and HHS, 2020). The Healthy Eating Index (HEI)-Toddlers-2020 is a dietary quality assessment tool that evaluates the extent to which toddler intake aligns with the *Dietary Guidelines for Americans, 2020–2025* (Pannucci et al., 2023). Applying the HEI-Toddlers-2020 to data from children aged 12–23 months in the National Health and Nutrition Examination Survey (2011–2018) revealed that average toddler dietary quality was 63% of the maximum score (Shams-White et al., 2023). This finding highlights the need for continued efforts to support parents in providing toddlers with nutritious diets that align with the *Dietary Guidelines for Americans*.

3.1.6 Contributing Factors to Difficulties Meeting Feeding Recommendations

The evidence on parent feeding practices during the first 2 years of life indicates that many parents have difficulty meeting evidence-based recommendations. Numerous studies have documented sociodemographic differences in feeding practices in the U.S. (CDC, 2022). Parents who are more socially disadvantaged tend to be less likely to meet the feeding recommendations (Chiang et al., 2023; Perrin et al., 2014; Wen et al., 2014). Many of these differences can be attributed to social and environmental inequities that impact access to the resources that caregivers need to meet infant and toddler feeding recommendations (Dixon et al., 2012). Policy, systems, and environmental (PSE) change strategies are essential to advancing health equity (Cohen et al., 2023; Kumanyika, 2019). For example, expanding access to paid caregiving leave, increasing housing and nutrition security, and increasing regulations on commercial infant formula marketing are PSE strategies that could have direct and indirect effects on parents' abilities to meet infant and toddler feeding recommendations (Kracht et al., 2024; Rollins et al., 2023). Given that PSE strategies typically take a long time to implement, and the continued importance of individualized support, PSE strategies should be implemented alongside strategies that increase individual and family resilience to stressors that limit parents' abilities to meet infant and nutrition feeding recommendations (Henry et al., 2015; Herman et al., 2022).

3.1.7 Information Behavior as a Modifiable Factor in Infant and Toddler Feeding

Both theory and research suggest that there are modifiable aspects of parenting behavior that could address some of the mechanisms through which social disadvantage influences child dietary intake and associated health outcomes (Wen et al., 2022). Parents' information behavior is one area of opportunity to support responsive parenting behaviors and nutritious child feeding practices. Many parents express interest in learning about positive parenting approaches and want more information to guide their parenting behaviors (Zero to Three & Bezos Family Foundation, 2016). Prior work has indicated that parents receive sometimes conflicting advice about infant and toddler nutrition from relatives, friends, health professionals, media sources (Carruth & Skinner, 2001; Matvienko-Sikar et al., 2018; McInnes et al., 2013; Savage et al., 2016; Sutter et al., 2018), and even directly from food packaging, such as formula canisters (Appleton et al., 2020). A few studies have explored how parents' sociodemographic characteristics influence information seeking for infant nutrition information (De Rosso et al., 2022; Quintero et al., 2023; Sutter et al., 2018). Findings generally suggest that parents who are more socially disadvantaged receive less total information and lower quality information than parents who are more socially advantaged. These findings underscore the importance of centering health equity and social justice when developing strategies for disseminating information about infant and toddler nutrition (Kumanyika, 2019).

As the evidence-based recommendations for infant and toddler nutrition continuously evolve, so too does the technology that parents may use to obtain information. Rapid changes in the digital information landscape, including social media platforms and features, artificial intelligence, and connected devices demand new and ongoing research on parents' information needs and preferences (Detopoulou et al., 2023; Doub et al., 2016a, b). Additional research on parents' information behavior is needed to inform the ongoing development and equitable dissemination of evidence-based parenting information (Hall & Bierman, 2015; McCatharn et al., 2021).

Information behavior has a long history of interdisciplinary research, but conceptual models that are commonly applied in the field of information science have yet to be extensively applied to studies investigating parenting behaviors, including infant and toddler feeding (Greyson, 2017; Kubb & Foran, 2020). When theory is applied, scholars tend to draw on traditional health behavior theories, that, while useful, have some limitations in terms of the research questions and hypotheses that they can motivate regarding information behavior (Greyson & Johnson, 2016). Interdisciplinary research that integrates concepts across fields specializing in health and human development and information science could generate insights into parents' information behavior. These insights could inform interventions that aim to increase alignment between parenting behavior and evidence-based recommendations.

3.1.8 Conceptual Model of Information Behavior

Figure 3.1 displays a new conceptual model of information behavior that integrates health behavior theories with conceptual models and frameworks from the field of information science. The conceptual model of information behavior is organized as a system. The conceptual model makes a series of testable predictions about whether and how individuals seek, process, use, and evaluate information, influenced by their needs, motivations, capacity, and the surrounding socioecological context and information environment. The conceptual model can be broadly applied to any information need, meaning any perceived gap in knowledge, interest, or curiosity (Given et al., 2023, pp. 1–18). The model is also valence free and can predict information behaviors that could be perceived as both positive and negative. For example, the model is equally suited to make predictions about obtaining evidence-based

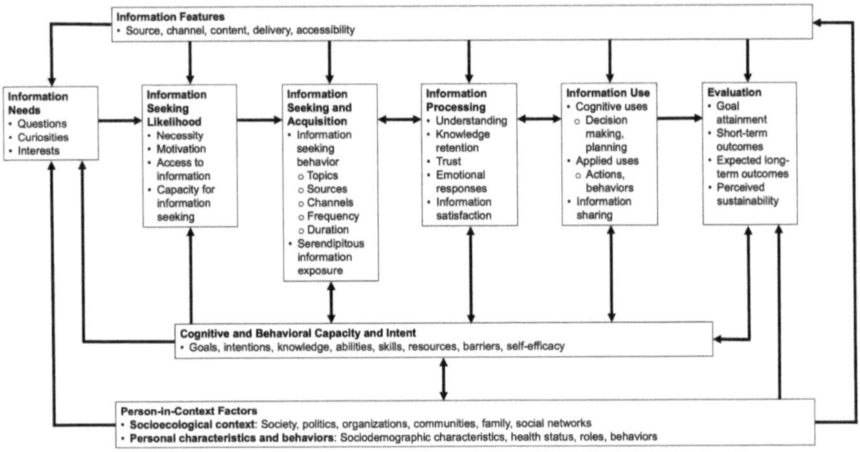

Fig. 3.1 Conceptual model of information behavior. *Note.* Bolded terms specify the model constructs. Bulleted terms specify example variables from each construct. Arrows specify the hypothesized associations between model constructs. Double arrows specify reciprocal associations

information as for obtaining misinformation. This new conceptual model contributes to an extant body of literature in the field of information science in which scholars synthesize existing models to make predictions about information behavior processes that can be tested and refined through empirical studies (Agarwal, 2022; Given et al., 2023, pp. 141–156). The remainder of this section describes the constructs and associations in the model.

3.1.8.1 Information Needs and Information Seeking Likelihood

Information needs can be defined as questions, curiosities, or interests that have personal or professional origins (Afzal, 2017; Dervin, 1998). Information needs often serve as a catalyst for new information behaviors and refer to gaps in knowledge that someone wants or needs to fill (Afzal, 2017; Dervin, 1998). As depicted in the model, information needs are influenced by information features, person-in-context factors, and cognitive and behavioral capacity and intent. For example, a person may serendipitously come across a topic they had not encountered before, which could spark a new information need. In digital information seeking contexts (e.g., search engines, social media platforms), search results, advertisements, and promoted content are often based on prior user behavior, thereby increasing the likelihood of serendipitous information exposure to previously searched topics or products (Lee & Cho, 2020). Parents of newborn infants are more likely to have information needs regarding establishing breastfeeding and/or choosing and preparing infant formula, whereas parents of toddlers are more likely to have information needs regarding meals, snacks, and picky eating.

Information needs are proposed to directly predict *information seeking likelihood,* which is the propensity for intentional information seeking. If there is no information need, a person is not likely to intentionally seek out information on a topic. Information needs that are time sensitive and serious, such as identifying symptoms of an allergic reaction after a child accidentally consumes a potentially allergenic food, are more likely to prompt a swift search. This proposed association is consistent with the Health Belief Model, which proposes that the perceived severity of a problem predicts action (Rosenstock, 1974). Information seeking likelihood directly predicts information seeking and acquisition, which includes intentional information seeking behavior and serendipitous information exposure. For example, parents who have access to many informational resources and a high capacity for seeking information (e.g., high health literacy) along with high necessity and/or motivation may be more likely to intentionally seek out information compared to those with access to fewer information resources and low capacity (e.g., low health literacy), especially if they also have low necessity and/or motivation (Morrison et al., 2019).

3.1.8.2 Information Seeking and Acquisition, Information Processing, and Information Use

Information seeking and acquisition, information processing, and information use are proposed to have sequential and reciprocal influences. While this process is common to most existing models of information behavior, the variables within each construct are numerous and the associations among them have yet been fully elucidated (Case & O'Connor, 2016; Sharot & Sunstein, 2020). *Information processing* refers to cognitive and affective processes that individuals experience to learn from and make sense of information. For example, understanding, trust, emotional reactions, and information satisfaction. Nahl's (2007) social-biological framework offers an in-depth analysis of the effects of emotions and other cognitive processes during information processing. The satisficing principal suggests that individuals iteratively engage in decision-making processes to decide whether or not they need more information (Winter, 2000). During infancy and toddlerhood, some information needs are finite, whereas others are ongoing. For example, a parent who is curious about when to start nighttime weaning from breastmilk or infant formula may have a relatively finite information need, whereas a parent looking for recipe ideas while introducing solid foods may engage in ongoing information searches.

Breakout Box 3.1: A Parent's Perspective

As a first-time mother of a three-month-old, I have spent my fair share of time researching infant nutrition to prepare myself for parenthood. In today's world, I have virtually every fact or piece of advice at my fingertips; a quick Internet search answers any question I may have. The difficulty of learning about infant nutrition, therefore, is not in accessing information, but in deciphering what information is accurate and valuable for my specific situation. If I am seeking an immediate answer to a simple question, I will often turn to the Internet, where I am met with a plethora of websites, blogs, and papers. When sorting through this vast array of information, I seek to find articles with clinically backed evidence and try to avoid old wives' tales or generational advice. In other words, I steer clear of blog posts from mothers offering personal anecdotes, as oftentimes what works for one family may not be what is recommended for the general public. I also seek to find consistency across articles by ensuring that what I'm reading lines up with what I already know to be true. When faced with too many conflicting pieces of evidence, however, I will always turn to my pediatrician. That way, if something were to go wrong, I have access to a professional who is aware of my actions and knows what possible causes/implications may be.

Dr. Hepworth would point out that many young parents turn to the Internet for information regarding their infant's nutrition, oftentimes out of curiosity over simple matters, yet sometimes for important concerns or urgent answers. While it is true that Internet searches are much quicker and cheaper than speaking with a professional, not all advice on the Internet is based on research. For this reason, parents must know when it is okay to seek answers from the Internet and when they should turn directly to a trusted professional.

— Mother of an infant

Information use has been relatively understudied compared to information seeking and acquisition to date, although the body of evidence is growing (Given et al., 2023). This is a critical gap because behavioral outcomes are often what researchers and health professionals are most interested in predicting (Greyson & Johnson, 2016). While there are many ways to conceptualize and define information use (Case & O'Connor, 2016; Spink & Cole, 2006), this conceptual model defines information use as cognitive uses (e.g., decision-making, planning), applied uses that involve actions and behaviors (e.g., making a purchase, using a new parenting approach), and information sharing (e.g., sharing information with a co-parent or grandparent). Examples of information use relevant to infant and toddler nutrition include decision-making about breastfeeding initiation and duration; when and how to introduce solid foods, including potentially allergenic foods; planning grocery lists for snacks and meals; purchasing specific brands of foods/beverages and feeding accessories (e.g., highchair, utensils); sharing information with a family relative; or using a new parenting strategy to respond to picky eating behaviors.

3.1.8.3 Evaluation

Evaluation occurs after individuals use (or do not use) the information that they obtained and processed. Critical self-reflection is considered an essential aspect of the learning process in adults (Mezirow, 1990). Evaluation is included in many existing models of information behavior such as Kuhlthau's information search process (Kuhlthau, 2004) and Dervin's sense-making theory (Dervin, 1998). Evaluation includes self-appraisals of whether the individual met their original goal, short-term and expected long-term outcomes associated with information use, and the perceived sustainability of the efforts required to achieve those outcomes. Person-in-context factors are proposed to directly affect evaluation because they influence an individual's capacity to engage in critical self-reflection; social norms regarding goal attainment (i.e., what is "good enough"); perceptions of desirable short- and long-term outcomes; and the conditions that impact sustainability (e.g., financial resources, social support).

Evaluation is proposed to be reciprocally associated with cognitive and behavioral capacity and intent. The extent to which individuals engage in intentional evaluation processes may vary depending on the original goal and associated information need. For example, parents who were seeking information on an infant feeding product (e.g., bib, spoon, and cup) may only briefly reflect on their purchasing behavior outcomes, whereas a parent who was seeking information on parenting strategies that decrease child food rejections at mealtimes may need to engage in a longer and more iterative period of critical self-reflection. The association is reciprocal because prior lived experiences, including emotions and physiological responses, can influence how individuals perceive new experiences (Jamieson et al., 2018). Ultimately, evaluation contributes to cognitive and behavioral capacity and intent, which in turn influences person-in-context factors, including individual-level behaviors. For example, a parent who tried a new breastfeeding position and evaluated it as comfortable, effective, and sustainable could then experience an increase in breastfeeding self-efficacy and thereby increase their breastfeeding duration.

3.1.8.4 Information Features

Information features are proposed to directly influence information needs, information seeking likelihood, information seeking and acquisition, information processing, information use, and evaluation. One of the most important information features is the content of the information itself. A fundamental example is that if information does not exist on a topic, or it is not accessible, a person will not be able to acquire that information. Considering information source as an information feature (e.g., whether the source is a friend, relative, or healthcare provider), social networks influence intentional information seeking and serendipitous exposure through social relationship dynamics such as homophily and social capital (Lin, 2002; McPherson et al., 2001). Considering information channel as an *information feature* (e.g., book, website, social media platform), multiple information science frameworks propose that some channels have more appeal than others, such as Uses and Gratifications Theory (Ruggiero, 2000), the Technology Acceptance Model (Davis, 1989), and the Unified Theory of Acceptance and Use of Technology (Venkatesh et al., 2016). For example, social media platforms and mobile applications often include features that motivate users to consistently use that channel (Sun & Zhang, 2021). Person-in-context factors also influence preferences for certain information sources (Doub et al., 2015; Doub et al. 2016a, b). Parents are likely to seek information about infant and toddler nutrition from accessible and preferred sources that meet their information needs.

3.1.8.5 Person-in-Context Factors

The conceptual model of information behavior incorporates Bronfenbrenner's (1977) ecological systems theory and asserts that individuals are embedded within larger contexts that influence all aspects of life, including information behavior. Contextual factors are integral to many existing conceptual models of information behavior (Johnson, 2003). For example, the comprehensive model of information seeking (Johnson & Case, 2012) and Savolainen's model for everyday information seeking (Savolainen & Thomson, 2022). Person-in-context factors include socio-ecological context (e.g., societies, political environments, organizations, families, and social networks) and personal characteristics and behaviors. Personal characteristics and behaviors include individual-level traits such as sociodemographic characteristics (e.g., age, gender, education, income, race, and ethnicity); health status (e.g., mental and physical health symptoms and diagnoses); and behaviors (e.g., parenting behaviors, personal dietary intake, and child feeding practices). Personal characteristics and behaviors also include an individual's role(s), particularly as the role relates to the information need. For example, whether the information need is personal or professional, and whether someone is seeking information for themselves or on behalf of someone else (i.e., surrogate information seeking; Kubb & Foran, 2020). Some information needs regarding infant and toddler nutrition can be conceptualized as surrogate searches on behalf of the child (e.g., symptoms of an allergic reaction to food), whereas other information needs are personal needs for the parent themselves (e.g., how to respond to challenging mealtime behaviors). For individuals who create content (e.g., public health professionals), the target audience's role is important to consider because it impacts the context in which the information will be processed and applied.

Person-in-context factors are proposed to directly affect information needs and have reciprocal associations with cognitive and behavioral capacity and intent. These associations are consistent with the health belief model (Rosenstock, 1974). In the context of infant and toddler feeding, person-in-context factors affect the perceived relevance and urgency of different child feeding topics; a parent's goals and intentions for their child feeding behaviors; the amount of motivation and time they have to obtain information; and the informational resources that they have access to. Person-in-context factors are also proposed to directly influence the nature and content of information (i.e., information features) as individuals and systems generate information (Savolainen, 2019).

3.1.8.6 Cognitive and Behavioral Capacity and Intent

Cognitive and behavioral capacity and intent are proposed to directly predict information needs and have reciprocal associations with information seeking likelihood, information seeking and acquisition, information processing, information use, and evaluation. This process is consistent with numerous health behavior theories, including Bandura's social cognitive theory (Bandura, 2001), the theory of planned behavior (Ajzen, 2012), and the transtheoretical model of behavior change (Prochaska & Velicer, 1997). In the context of child feeding, cognitive and behavioral capacity and intent refers to a parents' feeding goals and their ability to fulfill those goals based on their knowledge, skills, and resources. Recalling the reciprocal link between cognitive and behavioral capacity and intent and person-in-context factors, the conceptual model of information behavior proposes that humans can modify at least some aspects of their individual and collective lived experiences through information processing and use. For example, when qualifying parents learn about the Special Supplemental Nutrition Program for Women, Infants, and Children (WIC) program (information processing) and enroll and participate in WIC (information use), they gain access to tangible nutrition support (i.e., food package benefits) and educational programming that can increase parents' knowledge and skills related to nutritious child feeding practices (cognitive and behavioral capacity and intent). There is evidence that WIC program participation has intergenerational benefits on person characteristics, including improving maternal diet during pregnancy, child diet quality, and child cognitive development (Caulfield et al., 2022). These findings lend support to the proposed associations in the conceptual model.

3.1.9 Future Directions for Research Using the Conceptual Model of Information Behavior

The conceptual model of information behavior can inform future research on numerous information behavior topics, including on parents' information behavior regarding infant and toddler nutrition. Researchers frequently use quantitative surveys (i.e., questionnaires) to describe information behavior (Given et al., 2023, pp. 200–204). Surveys are useful for quantifying specific variables (e.g., the percentage of a population has searched for a specific topic) and for testing associations among variables (e.g., the association between health literacy and information source use). Researchers also commonly use qualitative methodologies such as interviews and focus groups to investigate information behavior, particularly when the research questions are focused on *why* and *how* a population engages with information (Given et al., 2023, pp. 204–210). Qualitative studies can be especially informative when investigating information use because of the large number of factors that contribute to how, when, and why information is applied (Case & O'Connor, 2016). Experimental studies that manipulate information behavior (e.g., randomized controlled trials) are also needed to generate causal evidence that reveals the mechanisms through information behavior affects parents' abilities to meet the evidence-based recommendations for infant and toddler nutrition (Obbagy et al., 2022). Descriptive and explanatory research studies can use the conceptual model of information behavior to identify constructs and variables to investigate and to generate hypotheses about their associations.

3.1.10 Empirical Study Aims and Objectives

Informed by the conceptual model of information behavior, the authors conducted a cross-sectional survey to describe first-time parents' information behavior regarding infant and toddler nutrition. We aimed to describe multiple variables within information need; information seeking and acquisition; information processing; and information use. Additionally, we tested the hypothesis that information satisfaction and affective responses would be associated with information use. The objective was to generate insights into parents' information behavior that can guide the dissemination of evidence-based guidance for infant and toddler nutrition.

3.2 Methods

First-time parents whose only or oldest child was ≤24 months old were recruited to complete a ~20-min online survey administered via *Qualtrics* (Provo, UT) about their experiences obtaining information about infant and toddler nutrition. Data were collected between February 06, 2018 and February 22, 2018. A commercial participant recruitment service, Research Now SSI (currently Dynata; https://www.dynata.com) recruited participants into the study from their online survey panel database of adults (≥ 18 years old) who resided in the United States and spoke English. To be eligible to participate, individuals had to consent to study participation, self-identify as a first-time parent of an only or oldest child ≤24 months old, and endorse remembering trying to get advice or information regarding infant or toddler nutrition topics in the past 30 days. All study procedures were reviewed by the Pennsylvania State University Office for Research Protections and were determined to be exempt.

3.2.1 Participant Sampling Approach

Participants were recruited using a purposive, quota-based convenience sampling approach (Campbell et al., 2020). Recruitment was targeted to promote an equitable representation of parents with infants in the following age ranges: 0–5 months, 6–11 months, 12–17 months, and 18–24 months. These age ranges, respectively, correspond to feeding stages: milk feeding period, introduction to solid foods, transition to the "adult" diet, and transition to structured meals and snacks (Pérez-Escamilla et al., 2017). Recruitment was also purposively targeted to promote an equitable representation of parents with annual household incomes in the following income ranges (Semega et al., 2017): Less than $25,000, $25,000 to $44,999, $45,000 and $74,999, $75,000 to $119,999, and over $120,000. Annual household income was selected as a sampling characteristic because children under age 2 years who live in lower-income households tend to have a higher risk of obesity in childhood and adolescence (Lee et al., 2014). Lastly, women and men were recruited with a goal of recruiting approximately 75% mothers and 25% fathers. This recruitment goal reflected the unique role that mothers have in infant feeding during the first 2 years of life, particularly through breastfeeding, and balancing an interest in including fathers with budget and time considerations for the survey. Fathers have been underrepresented in research on parents' feeding behavior with an average representation of 17% (Davison et al., 2016).

3.2.2 Measure Development Pilot Research

In order to develop the survey instrument for the current study, the first author (ADH) developed and tested study-specific measures in a two-phase pilot study that included qualitative semi-structured interviews (Whiting, 2008) and cognitive interviewing (Beatty & Willis, 2007). This qualitative approach to survey instrument development is consistent with recommendations for developing surveys with high measurement validity (Rattray & Jones, 2007). Pilot study procedures were reviewed by the Penn State University Office of Research Protections and determined to be exempt.

First, ADH conducted semi-structured interviews with parents of children under age 2 years (n = 7, 5 mothers, 2 fathers). The interviews explored concepts and processes from the conceptual model of information behavior in the context of infant and toddler nutrition. Each interview lasted ~60 min. Results informed the variables that were assessed in the survey and the phrasing of study-specific items.

Next, ADH programmed the survey in Qualtrics and iteratively modified the full survey to improve the clarity and flow of the instrument using cognitive interviewing with a separate group of parents of children under age 2 years ($n = 14$, 13 mothers, 1 father). The first participant completed the survey live during a telephone interview by reading each question and response option aloud. All other participants completed the survey independently online prior to a semi-structured telephone interview within 24-h of completing the survey. Interviews focused on the clarity of the survey items and response options and the extent to which the survey captured participants' lived experiences. Participants took ~30 min to complete the survey and each follow-up interview lasted ~25 min. Results led to further refinement of the survey items and response options. The following section details the finalized measures that were administered in the main study.

3.2.3 *Measures*

The following measures were administered to participants in the main study.

3.2.3.1 Participant Characteristics

Participants reported their demographic characteristics (gender, age, number of children, relationship to child, race, ethnicity, annual household income, current federal nutrition assistance program participation, marital status, education level, and employment status) and their child's gender and age. Parents of multiple children reported on their oldest child of 24 months of age or younger.

3.2.3.2 Information Seeking and Acquisition

Participants reported how often they had sought advice or information about infant and toddler nutrition in the past 30 days, when their most recent search was relative to completing the survey, how long they spent on their most recent search, the topics they searched for in the past 30 days, and the topic of their most recent search. For their most recent search only, participants reported what technology they used (if any), and all of the sources that they accessed to try to obtain information. Sources were presented in a random order to reduce order bias.

3.2.3.3 Information Processing

Participants reported their level of satisfaction with the advice or information they obtained during their most recent search. Participants responded to five items that assessed overall satisfaction (considering all sources that they tried), amount of information, level of detail, personalization, and actionability. All items were rated on a seven-point Likert scale with 1 = Not at all satisfied to 7 = Completely satisfied. A mean score was calculated and used in the analyses. The 5-item satisfaction measure had high internal consistency ($\alpha = 0.89$).

Participants also reported their affective responses to the information that they obtained during their most recent search. Specifically, participants endorsed whether or not the information that they obtained made them feel informed, reassured, empowered, motivated, overwhelmed, confused, frustrated, worried, and/or disappointed.

3.2.3.4 Information Use

Participants reported whether they had used the information that they obtained during their most recent search to make a decision, make a plan, make a purchase, prepare a recipe, use a new feeding approach, or use a new parenting approach. Response options were: "Yes," "No," "Not yet, but I plan to," or "N/A." The response options of "No," "Not yet, but I plan to," and "N/A" were combined in the analyses. Responses were also combined to indicate whether the participant had used the information in any way (i.e., any information use); in any cognitive way (i.e., to make a decision and/or make a plan); or in any behavioral way (i.e., to make a purchase, prepare a recipe, use a new feeding approach, and/or use a new parenting approach).

3.2.4 Statistical Analyses

Descriptive statistics were calculated for all study variables. Independent samples *t*-tests were conducted to test associations between information satisfaction and information use. Chi-square analyses were conducted to test associations between affective responses and information use. Results were considered statistically significant at $p < 0.05$. The few instances of missing data on single scale items ($n = 2$) were treated as missing.

3.3 Results

A total of 423 participants completed the survey. Participant demographic characteristics are reported in Table 3.1. The majority of participants were mothers (89%). Participants ranged in age from 18 to 54 years old and had a mean age of 28.4 years ($SD = 5.5$). Most participants had one child (92%) and were married (65%) or living with a romantic partner (25%). Nearly all participants were biologically related to the child they were reporting on (98%) and all but one participant were full-time

Table 3.1 Participant demographic characteristics in a sample of first-time parents of children ≤ 24 months old, United States, February 2018 ($N = 423$)

Characteristic	*n*	%
Parent gender		
Women	375	89%
Men	48	11%
Number of children[a]		
1 Child	389	92%
2 Children	34	8%
Parent race and ethnicity		
Asian, non-Hispanic	22	5%
Black or African American, non-Hispanic	40	9%
Black, Hispanic	2	< 1%
Hispanic or Latino alone	29	7%
White, non-Hispanic	299	71%
White, Hispanic	7	2%
Native American or Native Alaskan, non-Hispanic	3	1%
Two or more races endorsed	18	4%
Another race or ethnicity endorsed	3	1%
Annual household income		
Less than $24,999	81	19%
$25,000 to $44,999	126	30%
$45,000 and $74,999	110	26%
$75,000 to $119,999	75	18%
Over $120,000	31	7%
Federal Nutrition Assistant Program Participation		
WIC participant	108	26%
SNAP participant	67	16%
Marital status		
Married	270	64%
Single, living with romantic partner	106	25%
Single, never married, divorced, separated, or widowed	47	11%
Education level		
Less than high school	9	2%
High school diploma or GED	78	18%
Some college	104	25%

(continued)

Table 3.1 (continued)

Characteristic	*n*	%
Associate or bachelor's degree	175	41%
Graduate or advanced professional degree	57	14%
Employment status		
Employed, full-time	157	37%
Employed, part-time	60	14%
Full-time caregiver or stay-at-home parent	170	40%
Student	14	3%
Unemployed	19	5%
Other	3	1%
Child gender[a]		
Girls	195	46%
Boys	227	54%
Prefer not to answer	1	< 1%
Child age[a]		
0–5 months	97	23%
6–11 months	95	23%
12–17 months	118	28%
18–24 months	113	27%

[a] Participants with more than one child were asked to report on their oldest child of 24 months of age or younger

Note. SNAP = Supplemental Nutrition Assistance Program. WIC = Special Supplemental Nutrition Program for Women, Infants, and Children

residential parents. Despite efforts to recruit a balanced sample in terms of gender and household income, few fathers (11%) or parents with household incomes greater than $120,000 (7%) participated in this study. Over half (56%) of participants had incomes between $25,000 and $74,999. About one-quarter of participants were actively enrolled in WIC (26%). Recruitment efforts were successful in obtaining a balanced sample in terms of child age. Parents reported the following ages of their only or oldest child of 24 months of age: 0–5 months (23%), 6–11 months (23%), 12–17 months (28%), and 18–24 months (27%). The majority of participants identified as non-Hispanic White (71%) followed by non-Hispanic Black or African American (9%), Hispanic or Latino alone (7%), and non-Hispanic Asian (5%). A total of 51% of participants were employed either full-time (37%) or part-time (14%). Most parents who were not working reported being a full-time caregiver or stay-at-home parent (40%).

As shown in Fig. 3.2, participants frequently sought information about infant and toddler nutrition topics, most commonly multiple times per week in the past 30 days (n = 165, 39%). Participants most recent search occurred within 1 week for most participants ("one week ago or more recently," n = 336, 79%), and about half of

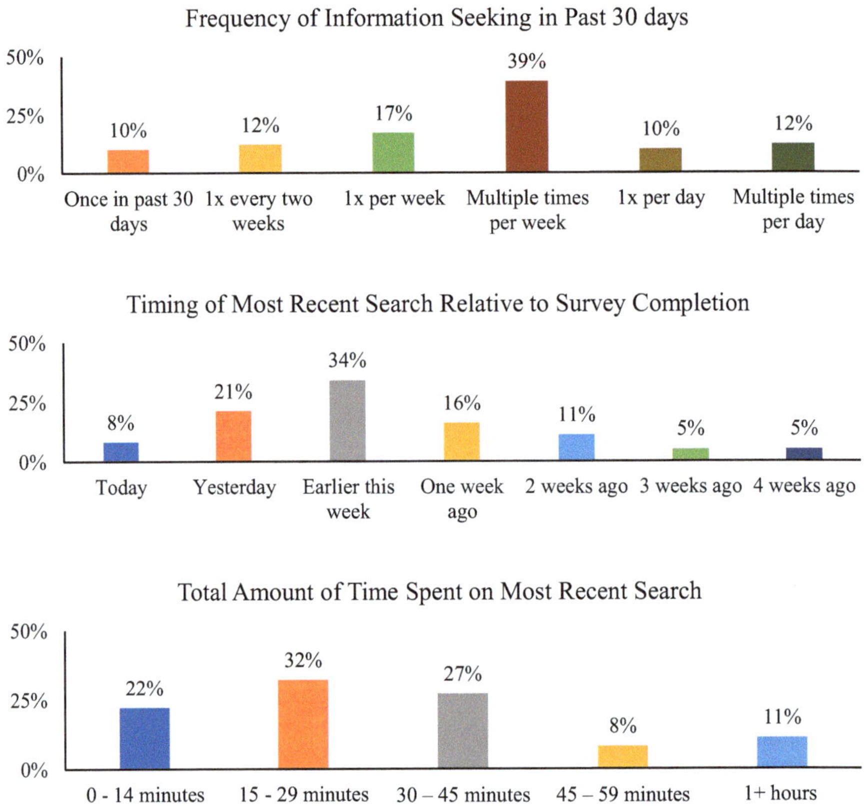

Fig. 3.2 Information seeking behaviors regarding infant and toddler nutrition among first-time parents of children ≤ 24 months old in the past 30 days, United States, February 2018 ($N = 423$)

participants spent less than 30 min on their search ("29 minutes or less," $n = 226$, 54%). Nearly all participants used technology during their search ($n = 396$, 94%), most commonly a smartphone ($n = 337$, 80%), followed by a computer ("laptop or desktop," $n = 122$, 29%), or tablet ($n = 56$, 13%).

The infant and toddler nutrition topics that participants searched for in the past 30 days and during their most recent search are shown in Table 3.2. Overall, the most common information need was for recipe or food preparation ideas, endorsed by 51% of participants ($n = 216$) as a topic searched in the past 30 days, and by 18% of participants ($n = 78$) as the topic of their most recent search. In the past 30 days, participants also sought information on child nutrition needs (44%), weight or child growth (41%), child behavior at mealtimes (36%), and breastfeeding (35%). During the most recent search, participants also commonly sought information on introducing solid foods ($n = 47$, 11%), picky eating ($n = 45$, 11%), and breastfeeding ($n = 38$, 9%).

The sources that participants accessed during their most recent search are reported in Table 3.3. Participants accessed an average of 3–4 sources during their

Table 3.2 Information needs regarding infant and toddler nutrition among first-time parents of children ≤ 24 months old, United States, February 2018 ($N = 423$)

	Last 30 Days		Most recent search	
Topic searched	n	%	n	%
Milk feeding topics				
Breastfeeding	149	35%	38	9%
Pumping breastmilk	112	27%	24	6%
Bottle feeding	112	27%	12	3%
Formula feeding	105	25%	11	3%
Weaning from milk	80	19%	15	4%
Adding cereal to the bottle	75	18%	17	4%
Complementary feeding topics				
Recipe or food preparation ideas	216	51%	78	18%
Introducing solid foods	130	31%	47	11%
Food or beverage products	115	27%	6	1%
Family meals	109	26%	8	2%
Baby-led weaning	72	17%	13	3%
Special occasion food or drink ideas	46	11%	5	1%
Child nutrition and health topics				
Child nutrition needs	185	44%	26	6%
Weight or growth	173	41%	25	6%
Child behavior at mealtimes	154	36%	18	4%
Picky eating	123	29%	45	11%
Food allergies or sensitivities	115	27%	25	6%
Other	15	4%	10	2%

most recent search ($M = 3.5$, $SD = 2.1$, range: 1–12). Several digital sources were highly endorsed, including search engines ($n = 225$, 53%), websites ($n = 221$, 52%), social media platforms ($n = 113$, 27%), and blogs ($n = 105$, 25%). Sources within participants' personal social networks were also highly endorsed, including family relatives ($n = 190$, 45%), pediatricians ($n = 134$, 32%), friends ($n = 120$, 28%), and co-parents ($n = 94$, 22%).

Participants reported relatively high satisfaction with the information they obtained during their most recent search ($M = 5.7$, $SD = 0.95$, range: 1.0–7.0). As shown in Fig. 3.3, participants also reported mostly positive affective responses to the information they obtained. Most participants applied the information they obtained in some way ($n = 365$, 86%). The most common applications were cognitive, including making a decision ($n = 276$, 65%) or making a plan ($n = 277$, 65%). Behavioral applications were also highly endorsed, particularly using a new feeding approach ($n = 181$, 43%), making a purchase ($n = 177$, 42%), and preparing a recipe ($n = 161$, 38%).

Participants' level of satisfaction with the information they obtained was positively associated with information use. Satisfaction was higher among participants who used the information in any way ($M = 5.81$, $SD = 0.88$) compared to those who

Table 3.3 Sources of information accessed during first-time parents' most recent search for infant and toddler nutrition information, United States, February 2018 ($N = 423$)

Source	n	%
Search engine (e.g., Google)[a]	225	53%
Followed link(s) from search engine results	169	40%
Only looked at featured search result	56	25%
Websites	221	52%
Family relative(s)	190	45%
Pediatrician	134	32%
Friend(s)	120	28%
Any social media platform[b]	113	27%
Facebook	81	19%
Pinterest	61	14%
Instagram	11	3%
Reddit	4	1%
Twitter	2	<1%
Blogs	105	25%
Co-parent	94	22%
Books (e.g., parenting books, cookbooks)	51	12%
WIC	34	8%
Hospital or other health care professional	30	7%
Online forums	29	7%
Apps	25	6%
Co-worker(s)	20	5%
Childcare provider(s)	15	4%
Handout from healthcare setting	10	2%

[a]Participants who endorsed using search engines were asked how they used the search engine results
[b]Participants who endorsed social media were asked to specific which social media platform(s) they accessed
Note. WIC = Special Supplemental Nutrition Program for Women, Infants, and Children

did not ($M = 5.20$, $SD = 1.21$), $t(66.96) = -3.66$, $p < 0.001$. Similarly, satisfaction was higher among participants who used the information in any cognitive way ($M = 5.87$, $SD = 0.83$) compared to those who did not ($M = 5.24$, $SD = 1.17$), $t(124.56) = -4.95$, $p < 0.001$, and higher among those who used the information in any behavioral way ($M = 5.81$, $SD = 0.89$) compared to those who did not ($M = 5.50$, $SD = 1.07$), $t(421)$, $p = 0.001$.

Some affective responses to information were associated with information use. Participants were more likely to use the information in any way if they felt informed, $\chi^2(1, N = 423) = 15.76$, $p < 0.001$ or motivated by the information they obtained, $\chi^2(1, N = 423) = 14.23$, $p < 0.001$. Conversely, participants were less likely to use the information in any way if they felt confused, $\chi^2(1, N = 423) = 9.00$, $p = 0.003$, worried, $\chi^2(1, N = 423) = 4.59$, $p = 0.03$, or disappointed by the information they

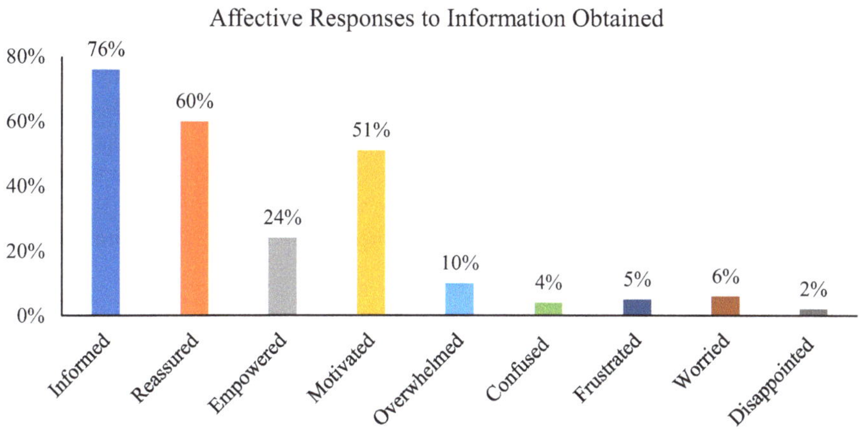

Fig. 3.3 Information processing and information use among first-time parents considering their most recent search for infant and toddler nutrition information, United States, February 2018 ($N = 423$)

obtained, $\chi^2(1, N = 423) = 7.34$, $p = 0.01$. Cognitive use was also more common when participants felt informed, $\chi^2(1, N = 423) = 16.24$, $p < 0.001$ or motivated by the information they obtained, $\chi^2(1, N = 423) = 14.80$, $p < 0.001$. Cognitive use was less common when participants felt confused, $\chi^2(1, N = 423) = 10.16$, $p = 0.001$, worried, $\chi^2(1, N = 423) = 4.54$, $p = 0.03$, or disappointed by the information they obtained, $\chi^2(1, N = 423) = 5.66$, $p = 0.02$. Behavioral use was more common when participants felt motivated, $\chi^2(1, N = 423) = 13.97$, $p < 0.001$) or empowered by the information they obtained $\chi^2(1, N = 423) = 4.91$, $p = 0.03$. There were no other statistically significant associations between affective responses and information use.

3.4 Implications

3.4.1 Implications for Understanding Family Resilience

Current statistics on parents' infant and toddler feeding practices in the U.S. indicate that parenting behaviors are frequently not aligned with the evidenced-based recommendations for breastfeeding, solid food introduction, potential allergen introduction, and dietary quality. Parents who are more socially disadvantaged tend to have greater challenges meeting infant and toddler nutrition recommendations, which contributes to health inequities throughout the lifespan (Dixon et al., 2012). Information behavior is a modifiable factor that could support nutritious feeding practices and improve child health if evidence-based information is disseminated equitably, and if the information fosters skill development and connects parents with meaningful support.

Parents' information behavior can support family resilience through increasing knowledge and connecting families to social support and material resources (Gonzalez et al., 2022). Lived experiences and knowledge about infant feeding can have intergenerational effects, as has been shown for breastfeeding (Woods Barr et al., 2021). Intentional information seeking and serendipitous information exposure provide parents with opportunities to develop their knowledge and attitudes about child feeding behaviors and can use the information they obtain to manage their basic resources (e.g., money, time) to meet their family's nutritional needs (Henry et al., 2015).

3.4.2 Implications for Practice

The goal of this empirical study was to describe variables within *information needs*, *information seeking and acquisition*; *information processing*; and *information use* from the new conceptual model of information behavior presented in this chapter. We also aimed to test the hypotheses that information satisfaction and affective responses would be associated with information use. Results showed that first-time parents regularly sought information about infant and toddler nutrition topics. Search topics reflected children's changing nutritional needs over the first 2 years of life. Recipe and food preparation ideas, introducing complementary foods, picky eating, and breastfeeding were among the most common information needs. Similar search topics were reported among parents in France, possibly suggesting commonality among parents in high-income countries (De Rosso et al., 2022). Public health professionals could intervene on parents' information behavior through informational campaigns that raise awareness of common infant feeding recommendations.

Most parents reported using a smartphone or computer during their search, and over half of searches included search engines (e.g., Google) and websites. Further, more than one-in-four parents reported using a social media platform. These results highlight the ongoing need and opportunity for professionals with expertise in infant nutrition and parenting behavior to create relevant, evidence-based digital content and/or direct parents to existing digital resources (Helm & Jones, 2016). Parents who follow social media influencers are highly likely to encounter information serendipitously, which can shape their knowledge, beliefs, and behaviors (Chee et al., 2023). As social media use and influencer culture continue to expand, incidental and serendipitous information exposure may supplement or replace intentional information seeking that is driven by specific needs (Reviglio, 2019). Parents must think critically about the information that they are exposed to on digital platforms to identify and avoid misinformation (Rowe & Alexander, 2022). Technology develops rapidly and some specific social media platforms that were not assessed or were not highly endorsed in this survey have become more popular in recent years, such as YouTube, Reddit, and TikTok (Auxier & Anderson, 2021). The percentage of parents using any given social media platform for information is dynamic. Health professionals should monitor current technology trends and adjust their information dissemination strategies accordingly.

Close social network connections, including family relatives, friends, and co-parents were highly endorsed as sources of information. Pediatricians were also endorsed by about one-in-three parents, and about one-in-ten parents reported getting information from WIC, the hospital, or another health care professional. Similar sources of infant and toddler nutrition information were reported among parents in France (De Rosso et al., 2022). Pediatricians, WIC, and other healthcare professionals such as registered dietitians and international board-certified lactation consultants have a critical role in disseminating evidence-based information. Health professionals can work directly with families and disseminate information through more wide-reaching media, like websites and social media.

As hypothesized, information satisfaction and affective responses were associated with information use. Parents who were more satisfied with the information that they obtained were more likely to use the information in anyway, for cognitive purposes, such as decision-making or planning, and behaviorally, such as to make a purpose or try a new feeding approach. Parents who felt informed or motivated were more likely to use the information in anyway and for cognitive purposes. Parents who felt motivated or empowered were more likely to use the information behaviorally. Feeling worried, confused, or disappointed was associated with a lower likelihood of using the information in any way and for cognitive purposes. These results are consistent with prior work on the effects of cognitive and affective processes on decision-making (Lerner et al., 2015) and purchasing behavior (Guo et al., 2020). Public health professionals can support family resilience by creating informative, motivating, and empowering content that conveys evidence-based recommendations for infant and toddler nutrition and disseminating it through commonly accessed and preferred channels.

3.5 Conclusion and Future Directions

Infants and toddlers rely on their parents and other primary caregivers to provide them with the nutrition they need for physical and cognitive development. In addition to programs that promote universal access to basic needs for food and housing, parents' child feeding behaviors can be supported by the broad dissemination and uptake of evidenced-based information on children's nutritional needs and child feeding behaviors that promote a nutritious diet and positive experiences with food. As technology and evidence-based recommendations continuously evolve, there is a need for ongoing research on parents' information behavior. Survey research could be strengthened by the development and validation of measures that assess parents' knowledge, self-efficacy, and behaviors regarding what and how they feed their children (Foti et al., 2020; Zimmer et al., 2023). Fundamental psychological aspects of information behavior (e.g., information satisfaction, information comprehension, trust) and affective responses to information also require additional measurement development and validation in order to improve scientific rigor and reproducibility (Flake & Fried, 2020). Qualitative studies can provide additional nuanced insights into parents' information behavior, particularly answering questions like how and why parents choose to use, or not use, information (Case & O'Connor, 2016).

The conceptual model of information behavior presented in this chapter synthesized health behavior theories that are commonly applied in public health research with theories and conceptual frameworks from the field of information science. By specifying key constructs, example variables, and the proposed mechanisms through which individuals find and apply information, this new conceptual model can foster precise and mechanistic research on parents' information behavior. Studies that identify parents' information preferences and factors that contribute to information use can guide ongoing efforts to align parenting behavior with evidence-based recommendations for infant and toddler nutrition.

Funding Acknowledgment This material is based upon work supported by the National Science Foundation (NSF) Graduate Research Fellowship Program (DGE1255832), the USDA Childhood Obesity Prevention Training Program (2011–67,001-30,117), and the Pennsylvania State University College of Health and Human Development Dissertation Research Endowment. Any opinions, findings, and conclusions or recommendations expressed in this material are those of the author(s) and do not necessarily reflect the views of the funding entities.

Discussion Questions

1. Choose one of the evidence-based recommendations for infant and/or toddler feeding that was presented in this chapter. How would you educate a parent/caregiver about this recommendation? Consider how the parent/caregiver's sociodemographic characteristics would impact your education plan.
2. What is another example of a health behavior where there is a gap between evidence-based recommendations and behavior? What are the evidence-based recommendations and what are the typical behaviors? How does information behavior influence the gap between recommendations and behavior in this new example?
3. Recall a time that you intentionally tried to obtain information on a topic and apply it to the conceptual model of information behavior. What new insights did you gain about your information behavior from applying this model to a personal example?
4. What is another theory or conceptual model from your academic field that could further explain and/or make predictions about information behavior? For example, how could attachment theory explain who people do—or do not—rely on as sources of information?

5. What two major constructs within the conceptual model of information behavior are most interesting to you? How are these constructs associated? What are 1–2 specific variables that are included within each construct? What is one research question and hypothesis that you could test using these variables that would be relevant to your area of interest?

References

Afzal, W. (2017). Conceptualisation and measurement of information needs: A literature review. *Journal of the Australian Library and Information Association, 66*(2), 116–138. https://doi.org/10.1080/24750158.2017.1306165

Agarwal, N. K. (2022). Integrating models and integrated models: Towards a unified model of information seeking behaviour. *Information Research, 27*(1). https://doi.org/10.47989/irpaper922

Ajzen, I. (2012). The theory of planned behavior. In P. A. M. V. Lange, A. W. Kruglanski, & E. T. Higgins (Eds.), *Handbook of theories of social psychology: Volume one* (pp. 438–459). SAGE.

Appleton, J., Fowler, C., Laws, R., Russell, C. G., Campbell, K. J., & Denney-Wilson, E. (2020). Professional and non-professional sources of formula feeding advice for parents in the first six months. *Maternal & Child Nutrition, 16*(3), e12942. https://doi.org/10.1111/mcn.12942

Auxier, B., & Anderson, M. (2021, April 7). Social media use in 2021. *Pew Research Center: Internet, Science & Tech.* https://www.pewresearch.org/internet/2021/04/07/social-media-use-in-2021/

Balantekin, K. N., Anzman-Frasca, S., Francis, L. A., Ventura, A. K., Fisher, J. O., & Johnson, S. L. (2020). Positive parenting approaches and their association with child eating and weight: A narrative review from infancy to adolescence. *Pediatric Obesity, 15*(10), e12722. https://doi.org/10.1111/ijpo.12722

Bandura, A. (2001). Social cognitive theory: An agentic perspective. *Annual Review of Psychology, 52*(1), 1–26. https://doi.org/10.1146/annurev.psych.52.1.1

Beatty, P. C., & Willis, G. B. (2007). Research synthesis: The practice of cognitive interviewing. *Public Opinion Quarterly, 71*(2), 287–311. https://doi.org/10.1093/poq/nfm006

Birch, L. L., & Doub, A. E. (2014). Learning to eat: Birth to age 2 y. *American Journal of Clinical Nutrition, 99*(3), 723S–728S. https://doi.org/10.3945/ajcn.113.069047

Black, M. M., & Aboud, F. E. (2011). Responsive feeding is embedded in a theoretical framework of responsive parenting. *Journal of Nutrition, 141*(3), 490–494. https://doi.org/10.3945/jn.110.129973

Bronfenbrenner, U. (1977). Toward an experimental ecology of human development. *American Psychologist, 32*(7), 513–531. https://doi.org/10.1037/0003-066X.32.7.513

Brown, A., & Harries, V. (2015). Infant sleep and night feeding patterns during later infancy: Association with breastfeeding frequency, daytime complementary food intake, and infant weight. *Breastfeeding Medicine, 10*(5), 246–252. https://doi.org/10.1089/bfm.2014.0153

Campbell, S., Greenwood, M., Prior, S., Shearer, T., Walkem, K., Young, S., Bywaters, D., & Walker, K. (2020). Purposive sampling: Complex or simple? Research case examples. *Journal of Research in Nursing, 25*(8), 652–661. https://doi.org/10.1177/1744987120927206

Carruth, B. R., & Skinner, J. D. (2001). Mothers' source of information about feeding their children ages 2 months to 54 months. *Journal of Nutrition Education, 33*(3), 143–147. http://dx.doi.org.ezaccess.libraries.psu.edu/10.1016/S1499-4046(06)60183-8

Carson, V., Lee, E.-Y., Hewitt, L., Jennings, C., Hunter, S., Kuzik, N., Stearns, J. A., Unrau, S. P., Poitras, V. J., Gray, C., Adamo, K. B., Janssen, I., Okely, A. D., Spence, J. C., Timmons, B. W., Sampson, M., & Tremblay, M. S. (2017). Systematic review of the relationships between physical activity and health indicators in the early years (0–4 years). *BMC Public Health, 17*(5), 854. https://doi.org/10.1186/s12889-017-4860-0

Case, D. O., & O'Connor, L. G. (2016). What's the use? Measuring the frequency of studies of information outcomes. *Journal of the Association for Information Science and Technology, 67*(3), 649–661. https://doi.org/10.1002/asi.23411

Caulfield, L. E., Bennett, W. L., Gross, S. M., Hurley, K. M., Ogunwole, S. M., Venkataramani, M., Lerman, J. L., Zhang, A., Sharma, R., & Bass, E. B. (2022). *Maternal and child outcomes associated with the special supplemental nutrition program for women, infants, and children (WIC)*. Agency for Healthcare Research and Quality (US). http://www.ncbi.nlm.nih.gov/books/NBK579797/

Centers for Disease Control and Prevention. (2022). *Breastfeeding report card United States, 2022*. Centers for Disease Control and Prevention. https://www.cdc.gov/breastfeeding/data/reportcard.htm

Chee, R. M., Capper, T. S., & Muurlink, O. T. (2023). The impact of social media influencers on pregnancy, birth, and early parenting experiences: A systematic review. *Midwifery, 120*, 103623. https://doi.org/10.1016/j.midw.2023.103623

Chiang, K. V., Hamner, H. C., Li, R., & Perrine, C. G. (2023). Timing of introduction of complementary foods—United States, 2016–2018. *Morbidity and Mortality Weekly Report, 69*, 1969–1973. https://doi.org/10.15585/mmwr.mm6953a1

Cohen, J. F. W., Stowers, K. C., Odoms-Young, A., & Franckle, R. L. (2023). A call for theory to guide equity-focused federal child nutrition program policy responses and recovery efforts in times of public health crisis. *Journal of the Academy of Nutrition and Dietetics, 123*(1), 15–28. https://doi.org/10.1016/j.jand.2022.07.016

D'Hollander, C. J., Keown-Stoneman, C. D. G., Birken, C. S., O'Connor, D. L., Maguire, J. L., Cohn, R., Lau, E., Laupacis, A., Parkin, P. C., Salter, M., Szatmari, P., Weir, S., Anderson, L. N., Borkhoff, C. M., Kowal, C., Mason, D., Abdurrahman, M., Anderson, K., Arbess, G., & Vandenberghe, H. (2022). Timing of introduction to solid food, growth, and nutrition risk in later childhood. *The Journal of Pediatrics, 240*, 102–109.e3. https://doi.org/10.1016/j.jpeds.2021.08.076

Daniels, L., Mallan, K. M., Fildes, A., & Wilson, J. (2015). The timing of solid introduction in an 'obesogenic' environment: A narrative review of the evidence and methodological issues. *Australian and New Zealand Journal of Public Health, 39*(4), 366–373. https://doi.org/10.1111/1753-6405.12376

Davis, F. D. (1989). Perceived usefulness, perceived ease of use, and user acceptance of information technology. *MIS Quarterly, 13*(3), 319–340.

Davison, K. K., Gicevic, S., Aftosmes-Tobio, A., Ganter, C., Simon, C. L., Newlan, S., & Manganello, J. A. (2016). Fathers' representation in observational studies on parenting and childhood obesity: A systematic review and content analysis. *American Journal of Public Health*, e1–e8. https://doi.org/10.2105/AJPH.2016.303391

De Rosso, S., Nicklaus, S., Ducrot, P., & Schwartz, C. (2022). Information seeking of French parents regarding infant and young child feeding: Practices, needs and determinants. *Public Health Nutrition, 25*(4), 879–892. https://doi.org/10.1017/S1368980021003086

Dervin, B. (1998). Sense-making theory and practice: An overview of user interests in knowledge seeking and use. *Journal of Knowledge Management, 2*(2), 36–46. https://doi.org/10.1108/13673279810249369

Detopoulou, P., Voulgaridou, G., Moschos, P., Levidi, D., Anastasiou, T., Dedes, V., Diplari, E.-M., Fourfouri, N., Giaginis, C., Panoutsopoulos, G. I., & Papadopoulou, S. K. (2023). Artificial intelligence, nutrition, and ethical issues: A mini-review. *Clinical Nutrition Open Science, 50*, 46–56. https://doi.org/10.1016/j.nutos.2023.07.001

Dixon, B., Peña, M.-M., & Taveras, E. M. (2012). Lifecourse approach to racial/ethnic disparities in childhood obesity. *Advances in Nutrition, 3*(1), 73–82. https://doi.org/10.3945/an.111.000919

Donovan, S. M., Aghaeepour, N., Andres, A., Azad, M. B., Becker, M., Carlson, S. E., Järvinen, K. M., Lin, W., Lönnerdal, B., Slupsky, C. M., Steiber, A. L., & Raiten, D. J. (2023). Evidence for human milk as a biological system and recommendations for study design—A report from

"breastmilk ecology: Genesis of infant nutrition (BEGIN)" working group 4. *The American Journal of Clinical Nutrition, 117*, S61–S86. https://doi.org/10.1016/j.ajcnut.2022.12.021
Doub, A. E., Levin, A., Heath, C. E., & LeVangie, K. (2015). Mobile app-etite: Consumer attitudes towards and use of mobile technology in the context of eating behaviour. *Journal of Direct, Data and Digital Marketing Practice, 17*(2), 114–129.
Doub, A. E., Small, M. L., & Birch, L. L. (2016a). A call for research exploring social media influences on mothers' child feeding practices and childhood obesity risk. *Appetite, 99*, 298–305. https://doi.org/10.1016/j.appet.2016.01.003
Doub, A. E., Small, M., Levin, A., LeVangie, K., & Brick, T. R. (2016b). Identifying users of traditional and internet-based resources for meal ideas: An association rule learning approach. *Appetite, 103*, 128–136. https://doi.org/10.1016/j.appet.2016.04.006
Ellis, J. M., Galloway, A. T., Webb, R. M., Martz, D. M., & Farrow, C. V. (2016). Recollections of pressure to eat during childhood, but not picky eating, predict young adult eating behavior. *Appetite, 97*, 58–63. https://doi.org/10.1016/j.appet.2015.11.020
Flake, J. K., & Fried, E. I. (2020). Measurement schmeasurement: Questionable measurement practices and how to avoid them. *Advances in Methods and Practices in Psychological Science, 3*(4), 456–465. https://doi.org/10.1177/2515245920952393
Foti, K., Perez, C. L., Knapp, E. A., Kharmats, A. Y., Sharfman, A. S., Arteaga, S. S., Moore, L., & Bennett, W. L. (2020). Identification of measurement needs to prevent childhood obesity in high-risk populations and environments. *American Journal of Preventive Medicine, 59*(5), 746–754. https://doi.org/10.1016/j.amepre.2020.05.012
Given, L. M., Case, D. O., & Willson, R. (2023). *Looking for information: Examining research on how people engage with information*. Emerald Group Publishing.
Gonzalez, C., Bollinger, B., Yip, J., Pina, L., Roldan, W., & Nieto Ruiz, C. (2022). Intergenerational online health information searching and brokering: Framing health literacy as a family asset. *Health Communication, 37*(4), 438–449. https://doi.org/10.1080/10410236.2020.1847445
Greyson, D. L. (2017). Health information practices of young parents. *Journal of Documentation*. https://doi.org/10.1108/JD-07-2016-0089
Greyson, D. L., & Johnson, J. L. (2016). The role of information in health behavior: A scoping study and discussion of major public health models. *Journal of the Association for Information Science and Technology, 67*(12), 2831–2841. https://doi.org/10.1002/asi.23392
Guo, J., Wang, X., & Wu, Y. (2020). Positive emotion bias: Role of emotional content from online customer reviews in purchase decisions. *Journal of Retailing and Consumer Services, 52*, 101891. https://doi.org/10.1016/j.jretconser.2019.101891
Hadley, C., Patil, C. L., & Gulas, C. (2010). Social learning and infant and young child feeding practices: Testing hypotheses about the transmission of child feeding information in Tanzania. *Current Anthropology, 51*(4), 551–560. http://dx.doi.org.ezaccess.libraries.psu.edu/10.1086/653998
Hall, C. M., & Bierman, K. L. (2015). Technology-assisted interventions for parents of young children: Emerging practices, current research, and future directions. *Early Childhood Research Quarterly, 33*, 21–32. https://doi.org/10.1016/j.ecresq.2015.05.003
Helm, J., & Jones, R. M. (2016). Practice paper of the academy of nutrition and dietetics: Social media and the dietetics practitioner: Opportunities, challenges, and best practices. *Journal of the Academy of Nutrition and Dietetics, 116*(11), 1825–1835. https://doi.org/10.1016/j.jand.2016.09.003
Henry, C. S., Sheffield Morris, A., & Harrist, A. W. (2015). Family resilience: Moving into the third wave. *Family Relations, 64*(1), 22–43. https://doi.org/10.1111/fare.12106
Herman, D. R., Blom, A., Tagtow, A., & Cunningham-Sabo, L. (2022). Implementation of an individual + policy, system, and environmental (I + PSE) technical assistance initiative to increase capacity of MCH nutrition strategic planning. *Maternal and Child Health Journal, 26*(1), 216–228. https://doi.org/10.1007/s10995-022-03435-0

Jamieson, J. P., Hangen, E. J., Lee, H. Y., & Yeager, D. S. (2018). Capitalizing on appraisal processes to improve affective responses to social stress. *Emotion Review, 10*(1), 30–39. https://doi.org/10.1177/1754073917693085

Janssen, X., Martin, A., Hughes, A. R., Hill, C. M., Kotronoulas, G., & Hesketh, K. R. (2020). Associations of screen time, sedentary time and physical activity with sleep in under 5s: A systematic review and meta-analysis. *Sleep Medicine Reviews, 49*, 101226. https://doi.org/10.1016/j.smrv.2019.101226

Johnson, J. D. (2003). On contexts of information seeking. *Information Processing & Management, 39*(5), 735–760. https://doi.org/10.1016/S0306-4573(02)00030-4

Johnson, J. D., & Case, D. O. (2012). *Health information seeking*. Peter Lang.

Johnson, S. L., Moding, K. J., & Bellows, L. L. (2018). Children's challenging eating behaviors: Picky eating, food neophobia, and food selectivity. In J. C. Lumeng & J. O. Fisher (Eds.), *Pediatric food preferences and eating Behaviors* (pp. 73–92). Academic Press. https://doi.org/10.1016/B978-0-12-811716-3.00004-X

Johnson, S. L., Gilley, S. P., & Krebs, N. F. (2022). Making every bite count: Best practices for introducing foods during the complementary feeding period. *The American Journal of Clinical Nutrition, 116*(1), 13–14. https://doi.org/10.1093/ajcn/nqac124

Kracht, C. L., Neshteruk, C. D., Moding, K. J., Rolke, L. J., Wagner, B. E., Kielb, E., Ferrante, M. J., Robinson, C., Keinsley, J., Colella, J., Speirs, K. E., & Luecking, C. T. (2024). Community-based diet and obesity-related policy, system, and environmental interventions for obesity prevention during the first 1000 days: A scoping review. *Obesity Reviews*. https://doi.org/10.1111/obr.13815

Krawiec, M., Fisher, H. R., Du Toit, G., Bahnson, H. T., & Lack, G. (2021). Overview of oral tolerance induction for prevention of food allergy—Where are we now? *Allergy, 76*(9), 2684–2698. https://doi.org/10.1111/all.14758

Kubb, C., & Foran, H. M. (2020). Online health information seeking by parents for their children: Systematic review and agenda for further research. *Journal of Medical Internet Research, 22*(8), e19985. https://doi.org/10.2196/19985

Kuhlthau, C. C. (2004). *Seeking meaning: A process approach to library and information services* (2nd ed.). Libraries Unlimited. http://swbplus.bsz-bw.de/bsz262326078inh.htm

Kumanyika, S. K. (2019). A framework for increasing equity impact in obesity prevention. *American Journal of Public Health, 109*(10), 1350–1357. https://doi.org/10.2105/AJPH.2019.305221

Langdon-Daly, J., & Serpell, L. (2017). Protective factors against disordered eating in family systems: A systematic review of research. *Journal of Eating Disorders, 5*(1), 12. https://doi.org/10.1186/s40337-017-0141-7

Lee, H., & Cho, C.-H. (2020). Digital advertising: Present and future prospects. *International Journal of Advertising, 39*(3), 332–341. https://doi.org/10.1080/02650487.2019.1642015

Lee, H., Andrew, M., Gebremariam, A., Lumeng, J. C., & Lee, J. M. (2014). Longitudinal associations between poverty and obesity from birth through adolescence. *American Journal of Public Health, 104*(5), e70–e76. https://doi.org/10.2105/AJPH.2013.301806

Lemaire, M., Huërou-Luron, I. L., & Blat, S. (2018). Effects of infant formula composition on long-term metabolic health. *Journal of Developmental Origins of Health and Disease, 9*(6), 573–589. https://doi.org/10.1017/S2040174417000964

Lerner, J. S., Li, Y., Valdesolo, P., & Kassam, K. S. (2015). Emotion and decision making. *Annual Review of Psychology, 66*(1), 799–823. https://doi.org/10.1146/annurev-psych-010213-115043

Lin, N. (2002). *Social capital: A theory of social structure and action*. Cambridge University Press.

Marshall, N. E., Abrams, B., Barbour, L. A., Catalano, P., Christian, P., Friedman, J. E., Hay, W. W., Hernandez, T. L., Krebs, N. F., Oken, E., Purnell, J. Q., Roberts, J. M., Soltani, H., Wallace, J., & Thornburg, K. L. (2022). The importance of nutrition in pregnancy and lactation: Lifelong consequences. *American Journal of Obstetrics and Gynecology, 226*(5), 607–632. https://doi.org/10.1016/j.ajog.2021.12.035

Masten, A. S. (2018). Resilience theory and research on children and families: Past, present, and promise. *Journal of Family Theory & Review, 10*(1), 12–31. https://doi.org/10.1111/jftr.12255

Matvienko-Sikar, K., Kelly, C., Sinnott, C., McSharry, J., Houghton, C., Heary, C., Toomey, E., Byrne, M., & Kearney, P. M. (2018). Parental experiences and perceptions of infant complementary feeding: A qualitative evidence synthesis. *Obesity Reviews, 19*(4), 501–517. https://doi.org/10.1111/obr.12653

McCatharn, J. M., Herbert, K. K., Wei, R., & Rowe, M. L. (2021). Circles of support: Exploring the 'where' and 'why' of parents' of infants information seeking behaviors. *Journal of Child and Family Studies*. https://doi.org/10.1007/s10826-021-02124-w

McInnes, R. J., Hoddinott, P., Britten, J., Darwent, K., & Craig, L. C. A. (2013). Significant others, situations and infant feeding behaviour change processes: A serial qualitative interview study. *BMC Pregnancy & Childbirth, 13*(1), 1–13. https://doi.org/10.1186/1471-2393-13-114

McPherson, M., Smith-Lovin, L., & Cook, J. M. (2001). Birds of a feather: Homophily in social networks. *Annual Review of Sociology, 27*, 415–444.

Meek, J. Y., Noble, L., & Section on Breastfeeding. (2022). Policy statement: Breastfeeding and the use of human milk. *Pediatrics, 150*(1), e2022057988. https://doi.org/10.1542/peds.2022-057988

Mezirow, J. (1990). *Fostering critical reflection in adulthood: A guide to transformative and emancipatory learning*. Wiley.

Moding, K. J., & Kielb, E. I. (2023). Conceptual considerations and methodological challenges to measuring food acceptance during infancy. *Current Nutrition Reports, 12*(3), 407–415. https://doi.org/10.1007/s13668-023-00480-1

Morrison, A. K., Glick, A., & Yin, H. S. (2019). Health literacy: Implications for child health. *Pediatrics in Review, 40*(6), 263–277. https://doi.org/10.1542/pir.2018-0027

Nahl, D. (2007). Social–biological information technology: An integrated conceptual framework. *Journal of the American Society for Information Science and Technology, 58*(13), 2021–2046. https://doi.org/10.1002/asi.20690

Obbagy, J., Raghavan, R., English, L. K., Spill, M. K., Bahnfleth, C. L., Bates, M., Callahan, E., Cole, N. C., Güngör, D., Kim, J. H., Kingshipp, B. J., Nevins, J. E. H., Scinto-Madonich, S. R., Spahn, J. M., Venkatramanan, S., & Stoody, E. (2022). Strengthening research that answers nutrition questions of public health importance: Leveraging the experience of the USDA nutrition evidence systematic review team. *The Journal of Nutrition, 152*(8), 1823–1830. https://doi.org/10.1093/jn/nxac140

Pannucci, T. E., Lerman, J. L., Herrick, K. A., Shams-White, M. M., Zimmer, M., Meyers Mathieu, K., Stoody, E. E., & Reedy, J. (2023). Development of the healthy eating index-Toddlers-2020. *Journal of the Academy of Nutrition and Dietetics, 123*(9), 1289–1297. https://doi.org/10.1016/j.jand.2023.05.013

Patterson, J. M. (2002). Understanding family resilience. *Journal of Clinical Psychology, 58*(3), 233–246. https://doi.org/10.1002/jclp.10019

Pattison, K. L., Kraschnewski, J. L., Lehman, E., Savage, J. S., Downs, D. S., Leonard, K. S., Adams, E. L., Paul, I. M., & Kjerulff, K. H. (2019). Breastfeeding initiation and duration and child health outcomes in the first baby study. *Preventive Medicine, 118*, 1–6. https://doi.org/10.1016/j.ypmed.2018.09.020

Pérez-Escamilla, R., Segura-Pérez, S., & Lott, M. (2017). Feeding guidelines for infants and young toddlers: A responsive parenting approach. *Healthy Eating Research*. http://healthyeatingresearch.org/research/feeding-guidelines-for-infants-and-young-toddlers-a-responsive-parenting-approach/

Perrin, E. M., Rothman, R. L., Sanders, L. M., Skinner, A. C., Eden, S. K., Shintani, A., Throop, E. M., & Yin, H. S. (2014). Racial and ethnic differences associated with feeding- and activity-related behaviors in infants. *Pediatrics, 133*(4), e857–e867. https://doi.org/10.1542/peds.2013-1326

Prochaska, J. O., & Velicer, W. F. (1997). The transtheoretical model of health behavior change. *American Journal of Health Promotion, 12*(1), 38–48. https://doi.org/10.4278/0890-1171-12.1.38

Quintero, S. M., Strassle, P. D., Londoño Tobón, A., Ponce, S., Alhomsi, A., Maldonado, A. I., Ko, J. S., Wilkerson, M. J., & Nápoles, A. M. (2023). Race/ethnicity-specific associations between

breastfeeding information source and breastfeeding rates among U.S. women. *BMC Public Health, 23*(1), 520. https://doi.org/10.1186/s12889-023-15447-8
Rattray, J., & Jones, M. C. (2007). Essential elements of questionnaire design and development. *Journal of Clinical Nursing, 16*(2), 234–243. https://doi.org/10.1111/j.1365-2702.2006.01573.x
Reupert, A., Straussner, S. L., Weimand, B., & Maybery, D. (2022). It takes a village to raise a child: Understanding and expanding the concept of the "village.". *Frontiers in Public Health, 10*, 756066. https://doi.org/10.3389/fpubh.2022.756066
Reviglio, U. (2019). Serendipity as an emerging design principle of the infosphere: Challenges and opportunities. *Ethics and Information Technology, 21*(2), 151–166. https://doi.org/10.1007/s10676-018-9496-y
Rollins, N., Piwoz, E., Baker, P., Kingston, G., Mabaso, K. M., McCoy, D., Neves, P. A. R., Pérez-Escamilla, R., Richter, L., Russ, K., Sen, G., Tomori, C., Victora, C. G., Zambrano, P., & Hastings, G. (2023). Marketing of commercial milk formula: A system to capture parents, communities, science, and policy. *The Lancet, 401*(10375), 486–502. https://doi.org/10.1016/S0140-6736(22)01931-6
Rosenstock, I. M. (1974). The health belief model and preventive health behavior. *Health Education Monographs, 2*(4), 354–386. https://doi.org/10.1177/109019817400200405
Rowe, S., & Alexander, N. (2022). Fighting nutrition and health misinformation: Enlisting the public's help. *Nutrition Today, 57*(1), 34. https://doi.org/10.1097/NT.0000000000000521
Ruggiero, T. E. (2000). Uses and gratifications theory in the 21st century. *Mass Communication and Society, 3*(1), 3–37. https://doi.org/10.1207/S15327825MCS0301_02
Savage, J. S., Fisher, J. O., & Birch, L. L. (2007). Parental influence on eating behavior: Conception to adolescence. *Journal of Law, Medicine & Ethics, 35*(1), 22–34. https://doi.org/10.1111/j.1748-720X.2007.00111.x
Savage, J. S., Neshteruk, C. D., Balantekin, K. N., & Birch, L. L. (2016). Low-income women's feeding practices and perceptions of dietary guidance: A qualitative study. *Maternal and Child Health Journal, 1–8*. https://doi.org/10.1007/s10995-016-2076-z
Savolainen, R. (2019). Modeling the interplay of information seeking and information sharing: A conceptual analysis. *Aslib Journal of Information Management, 71*(4), 518–534. https://doi.org/10.1108/AJIM-10-2018-0266
Savolainen, R., & Thomson, L. (2022). Assessing the theoretical potential of an expanded model for everyday information practices. *Journal of the Association for Information Science and Technology, 73*(4), 511–527. https://doi.org/10.1002/asi.24589
Scarpone, R., Kimkool, P., Ierodiakonou, D., Leonardi-Bee, J., Garcia-Larsen, V., Perkin, M. R., & Boyle, R. J. (2023). Timing of allergenic food introduction and risk of immunoglobulin e–mediated food allergy: A systematic review and meta-analysis. *JAMA Pediatrics, 177*(5), 489–497. https://doi.org/10.1001/jamapediatrics.2023.0142
Semega, J. L., Fontenot, K. R., & Kollar, M. A. (2017). *Income and poverty in the United States: 2016 (Current population reports P60–259)*. U.S. Census Bureau.
Shams-White, M. M., Pannucci, T. E., Lerman, J. L., Herrick, K. A., Zimmer, M., Meyers Mathieu, K., Stoody, E. E., & Reedy, J. (2023). Healthy eating Index-2020: Review and update process to reflect the dietary guidelines for Americans, 2020–2025. *Journal of the Academy of Nutrition and Dietetics, 123*(9), 1280–1288. https://doi.org/10.1016/j.jand.2023.05.015
Sharot, T., & Sunstein, C. R. (2020). How people decide what they want to know. *Nature Human Behaviour, 4*(1), Article 1. https://doi.org/10.1038/s41562-019-0793-1
Spill, M. K., Callahan, E. H., Shapiro, M. J., Spahn, J. M., Wong, Y. P., Benjamin-Neelon, S. E., Birch, L., Black, M. M., Cook, J. T., Faith, M. S., Mennella, J. A., & Casavale, K. O. (2019). Caregiver feeding practices and child weight outcomes: A systematic review. *The American Journal of Clinical Nutrition, 109*(Supplement_7), 990S–1002S. https://doi.org/10.1093/ajcn/nqy276
Spink, A., & Cole, C. (2006). Human information behavior: Integrating diverse approaches and information use. *Journal of the American Society for Information Science and Technology, 57*(1), 25–35. https://doi.org/10.1002/asi.20249
Sun, Y., & Zhang, Y. (2021). A review of theories and models applied in studies of social media addiction and implications for future research. *Addictive Behaviors, 114*, 106699. https://doi.org/10.1016/j.addbeh.2020.106699

Sutter, C., Fiese, B. H., Lundquist, A., Davis, E. C., McBride, B. A., & Donovan, S. M. (2018). Sources of information and support for breastfeeding: Alignment with Centers for Disease Control and Prevention strategies. *Breastfeeding Medicine, 13*(9), 598–606. https://doi.org/10.1089/bfm.2018.0056

Togias, A., Cooper, S. F., Acebal, M. L., Assa'ad, A., Baker, J. R., Beck, L. A., Block, J., Byrd-Bredbenner, C., Chan, E. S., Eichenfield, L. F., Fleischer, D. M., Fuchs, G. J., Furuta, G. T., Greenhawt, M. J., Gupta, R. S., Habich, M., Jones, S. M., Keaton, K., Muraro, A., & Boyce, J. A. (2017). Addendum guidelines for the prevention of peanut allergy in the United States: Report of the National Institute of Allergy and Infectious Diseases-sponsored expert panel. *The Journal of Allergy and Clinical Immunology, 139*(1), 29–44. https://doi.org/10.1016/j.jaci.2016.10.010

Totzauer, M., Escribano, J., Closa-Monasterolo, R., Luque, V., Verduci, E., ReDionigi, A., Langhendries, J.-P., Martin, F., Xhonneux, A., Gruszfeld, D., Socha, P., Grote, V., Koletzko, B., et al. (2022). Different protein intake in the first year and its effects on adiposity rebound and obesity throughout childhood: 11 years follow-up of a randomized controlled trial. *Pediatric Obesity, 17*(12), e12961. https://doi.org/10.1111/ijpo.12961

U.S. Department of Agriculture and U.S. Department of Health and Human Services. (2020). Dietary Guidelines for Americans, 2020-2025 (9th Edition).

U.S. Food & Drug Administration. (2023). *Food allergies*. U.S. Food & Drug Administration; FDA. https://www.fda.gov/food/food-labeling-nutrition/food-allergies

USDA and HHS. (2020). Infants and toddlers. In *Dietary guidelines for Americans, 2020–2025* (9th ed.). USDA and HHS. https://www.dietaryguidelines.gov

Venkatesh, V., Thong, J. Y., & Xu, X. (2016). Unified theory of acceptance and use of technology: *A synthesis and the road ahead. Journal of the Association for Information Systems, 17*(5), 328. https://doi.org/10.17705/1jais.00428

Venter, C., Warren, C., Samady, W., Nimmagadda, S. R., Vincent, E., Zaslavsky, J., Bilaver, L., & Gupta, R. (2022). Food allergen introduction patterns in the first year of life: A US nationwide survey. *Pediatric Allergy and Immunology, 33*(12), e13896. https://doi.org/10.1111/pai.13896

Ventura, A. K., & Whaley, S. E. (2022). Strategies to promote responsive bottle-feeding in WIC predict less frequent use of food to soothe and healthier weight status for infants with negative temperaments. *Pediatric Obesity, 17*(8), e12908. https://doi.org/10.1111/ijpo.12908

Wen, X., Kong, K. L., Eiden, R. D., Sharma, N. N., & Xie, C. (2014). Sociodemographic differences and infant dietary patterns. *Pediatrics, 134*(5), e1387–e1398. https://doi.org/10.1542/peds.2014-1045

Wen, X., Mi, B., Wang, Y., Taveras, E. M., & Bartashevskyy, M. (2022). Potentially modifiable mediators for socioeconomic disparities in childhood obesity in the United States. *Obesity, 30*(3), 718–732. https://doi.org/10.1002/oby.23379

Whiting, L. S. (2008). Semi-structured interviews: Guidance for novice researchers. *Nursing Standard (Royal College of Nursing (Great Britain): 1987), 22*(23), 35–40. https://doi.org/10.7748/ns2008.02.22.23.35.c6420

Winter, S. G. (2000). The satisficing principle in capability learning. *Strategic Management Journal, 21*(10/11), 981–996.

Woods Barr, A. L., Austin, D. A., Smith, J. L., & Schafer, E. J. (2021). "…[t]his is what we are missing": The value of communicating infant feeding information across three generations of African American women. *Journal of Human Lactation, 37*(2), 279–288. https://doi.org/10.1177/0890334421995078

Zero to Three, & Bezos Family Foundation. (2016). *Tuning in: Parents of young children speak up about what they think, know and need*. https://www.zerotothree.org/resource/national-parent-survey-report/

Zimmer, M., Obbagy, J., Scanlon, K. S., Gibbs, K., Lerman, J. L., Hamner, H. C., Pannucci, T., Sharfman, A., Reedy, J., & Herrick, K. A. (2023). Count every bite to make "every bite count": Measurement gaps and future directions for assessing diet from birth to 24 months. *Journal of the Academy of Nutrition and Dietetics, 123*(9), 1269–1279.e1. https://doi.org/10.1016/j.jand.2023.05.011

Chapter 4
Food, Eating Behavior, and Obesity Prevention

Ashlea Braun

To what extent can we exercise control over the foods we consume? How do we successfully change what we eat, and how can we ensure long-term success in this endeavor? While evidence has established that diet contributes to risk of and severity of outcomes associated with chronic diseases (Morze et al., 2020), consumption of foods known to be advantageous (e.g., fruits and vegetables) remains suboptimal while that of foods known to increase chronic disease risk [e.g., sugar-sweetened beverages (SSBs)] remains excessive. In 2009, an estimated 0.9% of adolescents and 2.2–3.5% of adults (men and women, respectively) consistently met the recommendation for fruit and vegetable consumption (Kimmons et al., 2009). This estimation has improved (e.g., 12.3% of adults met fruit recommendation and 10% met vegetable recommendation in 2019) (Lee, 2022); however, persistent insufficiency of fruit and vegetable consumption remains with much room for improvement. Similar trends are seen in other indicators of diet quality and consumption patterns. For example, per capita consumption of SSBs decreased across racial and ethnic groups from 2003 to 2018 (e.g., decreased from 81.6% to 72.7% among non-Hispanic White children and from 83.2% to 74.8% among non-Hispanic Black children) (Dai et al., 2021).

Food preferences and patterns of consumption are shaped in part by early life experiences and exposures (Hood et al., 2000; Scaglioni et al., 2018). Substantial attention has thus been directed at children, including school-based obesity prevention interventions, with mixed findings (e.g., such programs do not consistently

A. Braun (✉)
Hudson College of Public Health, University of Oklahoma Health Sciences
Oklahoma City, OK, USA

TSET Health Promotion Research Center, OU Health Stephenson Cancer Center
Tulsa, OK, USA
e-mail: Ashlea-Braun@ouhsc.edu

G. Welch et al. (eds.), *Stress, Resilience, and Healthy Relationships with Food and Family*, Emerging Issues in Family and Individual Resilience,
https://doi.org/10.1007/978-3-031-98937-7_4

demonstrate measurable effects on body mass index or measures of adiposity) (Hung et al., 2015). Evidence highlights the critical role of parental involvement in interventions (Sobol-Goldberg et al., 2013). Parental influences include child feeding (e.g., feeding styles) and the indirect influences of the parents' own food consumption patterns and eating behavior (Vaughn et al., 2018). Data from the Framingham Children's Study—a longitudinal study of childhood risk factors for cardiovascular disease (Moore et al., 1995)—demonstrated children whose parents had higher levels of disinhibition and dietary restraint had higher levels of body fat (Hood et al., 2000). Disinhibition and dietary restraint represent eating behaviors speculated to contribute to obesity risk, and include overeating in response to stimuli (e.g., stress) as well as a tendency to restrict food intake, respectively (Stunkard & Messick, 1985). Existing interventions targeting parents have had limited efficacy due to socioecological factors [e.g., obesogenic food environments rich in ultra-processed foods (UPF)], limiting parents' ability to implement recommendations (Norman et al., 2019; Ravikumar et al., 2022). In addition to the omnipresence of UPF, they offer convenience and practicality (Vidal et al., 2021). Barring drastic changes in macro-level influences, strategies must be established to support parental resiliency in order to break the cycle of dietary patterns conducive to the development of obesity and chronic disease.

4.1 Eating Behavior and the Risk of Chronic Illness and Obesity

Despite an enhanced understanding of the nutrient composition of foods and the advantages of consuming sufficient fruits, vegetables, whole grains, lean meats, and other nutrient-dense foods, habitual dietary patterns in the United States (US) remain suboptimal (Lee, 2022). The prevailing dietary pattern in the US has been and remains a Western Diet, characterized by heavy processing of foods rich in added sugars and fat (Adolph & Tilg, 2024), which has been implicated in obesity and related chronic illness (Cordain et al., 2005). Data from the National Health and Nutrition Examination Survey (NHANES) indicate that while modest improvements in diet quality have been observed over time, many in the US still have what are considered poor diets according to evidence-based guidelines (e.g., compliance with the US Dietary Guidelines) (Liu et al., 2021a), which are tied to conditions responsible for the majority of morbidity and mortality (e.g., cardiovascular disease) (Wang et al., 2021a). Thus, urgency exists to understand why diets in the US remain poor and address gaps that remain in fundamental characteristics of a healthy diet (i.e., fruit and vegetable consumption).

In addition to external factors (e.g., the food environment), individual-level variables such as the propensity for eating in response to emotional cues (i.e., emotional eating) influence the quantity and quality of foods one consumes, and these are further influenced by additional individual-level factors (e.g., depression) (Konttinen et al., 2019) as well as external factors (e.g., social networks). For example, Thomas and colleagues found that the frequency of overeating increases when individuals are exposed to more palatable foods in their environments (Thomas et al., 2011). Such individual-level patterns and approaches to consumption are often classified as eating behavior. Eating behavior constructs in adult populations include disinhibition, hunger, emotional eating, and cognitive restraint as measured by various versions of the Three Factor Eating Questionnaire (Stunkard & Messick, 1985); emotional eating, external eating, and retrained eating as measured by the Dutch Eating Behavior Questionnaire (van Strien et al., 1986); and others (Hunot et al., 2016; Marijn Stok et al., 2018). These traits have been implicated in the risk of and development of obesity. For example, disinhibition may be related to more hedonically driven food choices, contributing to overconsumption of foods that contribute to excess energy intake and, ultimately, risk of obesity (Bryant et al., 2019). Similarly, emotional eating may be related to the consumption of problematic food choices (e.g., fast food consumption), obesity, and depression (Dakanalis et al., 2023). These factors are of paramount importance when studying how individuals respond to and interact with obesogenic food environments. In addition, the experience of food insecurity is also likely to influence eating behavior (Goode et al., 2023). For example, Goode et al. (2023) found individuals utilizing the Supplemental Nutrition Assistance Program (SNAP) endorsed experiencing a loss of control when eating over worry of not having enough food. These experiences may be further moderated by the overarching food environment (Lorts et al., 2019). In response to such exposures and experiences, individuals may overeat when food is available, or set rules and restrictions around foods that can or cannot be consumed (Polivy et al., 2020), often represented by eating restraint. Eating restraint may promote a hyperfixation on food and food restrictions, particularly in those with a propensity toward disinhibition (Johnson et al., 2012), leading to disordered eating and obesity. However, it may also be protective if it enables individuals to exercise control in a flexible manner (Bryant et al., 2019) and may predict response to weight loss interventions (Papini et al., 2022). When eating restraint is done in a flexible manner, meaning foods associated with an increased risk of obesity (e.g., those with added sugars) can be consumed in small quantities, it may be most advantageous for mitigating the risk of diet-associated chronic disease, and facilitating this process may improve self-regulation of eating (Johnson et al., 2012).

Measures of eating behavior may be responsive to dietary or lifestyle intervention (De Leon et al., 2019), and may be a better behavioral target to facilitate improvements in health as opposed to diet alone (van Strien, 2018). Theory-driven interventions targeting behavior change demonstrate that eating behavior can be changed. Järvelä-Reijonen and colleagues found that an acceptance and commitment therapy intervention improves measures of eating behavior, including eating regulation and uncontrolled eating (Järvelä-Reijonen et al., 2018). However, the authors point out that no improvements in actual diet were observed, suggesting the need for specific dietary intervention in addition to addressing eating behavior. Indeed, certain dietary constituents (e.g., dietary fiber) present in various food groups (e.g., fruits and vegetables) may have unique influences on eating behavior due to specific biological effects. For example, emerging research suggests dietary fiber can modulate the gut microbiome and production of short-chain fatty acids, which have potential for neurological impacts (Goswami et al., 2018; Medawar et al., 2021). Thus, simultaneously encouraging adherence to evidence-based guidelines is an important element in interventions.

4.2 Bidirectional Relationship Between Food and Behavior

When contemplating how to modify behavior as it pertains to food and eating, the relationship between these two variables is often viewed as unidirectional: one must increase their motivation and change their behavior in order to modify their diet and improve their health (Satia et al., 2001). This perspective has limited the effectiveness of tested interventions, as exercising control over one's food choices in order to make substantial and clinically meaningful changes in diet is exceedingly difficult (Monteban et al., 2018; Spinelli & Monteleone, 2021). These are also influenced by internal factors that are shaped early in life (e.g., food preference) (Spahn et al., 2019), as well as those that are shaped over time (e.g., knowledge, attitudes) (Brecic et al., 2022). While motivation and related constructs (e.g., self-efficacy) are pertinent when examining and modifying human behavior, they are not the sole determinants that warrant consideration. Greater attention has been paid overtime to influences external to the individual that dictate these factors (Freedman et al., 2019; McLeroy et al., 1988). However, less attention has been paid to the individual-level factors that are influenced by ingested foods and beverages. That is, what impact does food have on our behavior?

Certain dietary constituents appear to be key candidates when considering the effects that food can have on behavior. One particular category of food that has emerged in recent years is UPF. Defined primarily by the Nova Food Classification System, UPF are defined as "industrial formulations typically with five or more and usually many ingredients. Such ingredients often include those also used in processed foods, such as sugar, oils, fats, salt, antioxidants, stabilizers, and preservatives. Ingredients only found in ultra-processed products include substances not commonly used in culinary preparations, and additives whose purpose is to imitate sensory qualities of (unprocessed or minimally processed) foods or of culinary preparations of these foods, or to disguise undesirable sensory qualities of the final product" (Monteiro et al., 2016). Commonly consumed UPF in the US include SSBs, snack foods, reconstituted meat products (e.g., chicken nuggets), and commercially prepared sweet foods (e.g., packaged cookies) (Juul et al., 2022). Many UPF contain ingredients that humans are innately drawn to consume (e.g., sugar, fat), as well as industrial additives that enhance the sensory experiences of foods, such as hydrogenated oils to improve texture, hydrolyzed vegetable proteins to improve flavor, high fructose corn syrup to increase sweetness, and caramel color to improve appearance (Tseng et al., 2022). Though these ingredients are safe to consume, they appear to render a food product that is ultimately hard to resist and foods rich in these ingredients appear associated with an increased risk of chronic disease (Neumann & Fasshauer, 2022). Recent work by Hall and colleagues demonstrates that, for example, diets comprised entirely of UPF lead to excessive ad libitum energy consumption as compared to unprocessed diets matched for calories and multiple nutrients and dietary fiber (Hall et al., 2019), suggesting consumption of certain foods contributes to changes in eating behavior and ongoing habitual consumption, ultimately influencing weight and overall health. The reasons for these impacts are not well known, but may include factors such as the soft texture of these foods or their ubiquity in food environments. These attributes are further compounded by the convenience and practicality UPF offer (Vidal et al., 2021). Further, UPF exposure and consumption may render neurobiological effects (Contreras-Rodriguez et al., 2022) that ultimately influence eating behavior, such as influencing reward processing. This potential is particularly concerning the earlier in life that the foods are introduced (De Amicis et al., 2022). At present, UPF make up the majority of energy intake for many US children (Wang et al., 2021b) and adults (Juul et al., 2022), their consumption has increased over time (Juul et al., 2022), and they may be disproportionally marketed toward high-risk populations (James et al., 2014; Leung et al., 2022).

While certain dietary constituents appear to harm health and negatively influence behavior, some are protective, and one candidate of interest is dietary fiber. Dietary fiber is not digested nor absorbed by the gastrointestinal tract, thus reaches the colon largely intact, and in some instances is fermented by the colonic microflora. In addition to advantageous attributes related directly to dietary patterns (e.g., dietary fiber is rich in plant foods which are generally less energy-dense than low-dietary fiber containing counterparts), dietary fiber may have influences on cognition and subsequently thoughts and behavior (e.g., food-related decision making) (Medawar et al., 2024). A potential mechanism by which dietary fiber can render these effects is via the colonic microbiome. Medawar and colleagues found that habitual dietary fiber intake is related to the presence of certain bacterial genera (e.g., *Parabacteroides*) and production of certain metabolites (e.g., short-chain fatty acids), which may influence measures of eating behavior via the TFEQ (e.g., disinhibition) through mechanisms not yet fully understood (Medawar et al., 2021). Animal models have also shown that dietary fiber interventions can alter preference for certain flavors (e.g., lessen the preference for sweet taste) (Bernard et al., 2019). Similar findings are seen in dietary fiber interventions targeting humans; however, these often enlist the use of supplements which do not afford all the benefits of consuming fiber-containing foods (e.g., nutrient density, high volume, calorie displacement) (Kaczmarczyk et al., 2012). Brief (i.e., 2-week) whole-food dietary fiber interventions have shown to improve short-term dietary fiber intake (Oliver et al., 2021). They may also alter the composition of microbial taxa present in the microbiome, and have the potential to modulate production of metabolites known to augment health (Koh et al., 2016), serving as a key contributor to communication between the brain and gut (Silva et al., 2020). Collectively, this evidence points to key dietary foci when trying to facilitate changes in eating behavior.

4.3 Parent and Child Eating: The Cycle of Dietary Patterns and Eating Behavior

The relationship between parental (e.g., maternal) dietary patterns and offspring health, eating behavior, and diet begins in utero (Liu, X. et al., 2021b; Miyake et al., 2023). In the nationwide prospective cohort study of 76,207 mother–infant dyads (the Japan Environment and Children's Study), Miyake and colleagues found that low maternal consumption of dietary fiber was associated with issues in child communication, fine motor, problem-solving, and personal-social skills (Miyake et al., 2023). Such effects appear to extend to child dietary consumption, with Spahn and colleagues finding evidence that specific foods consumed during pregnancy can transfer to and flavor amniotic fluid, increasing acceptance of these foods in infancy (Spahn et al., 2019). Other prenatal factors and/or birth outcomes render effects as well, with Boone-Heinonen and colleagues finding that infant birthweight (i.e., both low and high birthweight) is associated with energy consumption by children in the absence of hunger, particularly in the form of sweet foods (Boone-Heinonen et al., 2019).

Effects of maternal diet persist after birth via breastfeeding, feeding patterns, and indirect effects (e.g., behavioral modeling) (Lopez et al., 2018; Saltzman et al., 2016). Building upon in utero exposure, early introduction to the tastes of traditionally "healthy" foods (e.g., vegetables) via breastmilk may be an opportunity to improve acceptance of and preference for these foods later in life (Mennella et al., 2017). However, continued exposure to such foods is important. Data comparing formula-fed and breastfed infants demonstrate that repeated exposure to these foods after the introduction of solid foods and weaning is of paramount importance for acceptance (Forestell & Mennella, 2007). This can be done via gradual, repeated exposure (e.g., offering vegetables/vegetable purees) as infants transition to solid foods (Hetherington et al., 2015).

As children grow, they continue to be shaped by their food environments, and the consumption patterns of those around them. Specifically, the home food environment continues to influence child acceptance and consumption of healthy foods (Blanchette & Brug, 2005; Pearson et al., 2009). Raggio and colleagues found that among a population of school-aged children, intake of vegetables was determined in part by sensory characteristics (e.g., color and flavor) as well as patterns of consumption in the family environment. More specifically, children may have an innate dislike for the flavor attributes of vegetables (e.g., bitter taste); thus if preference for these foods is not cultivated via early life exposures (e.g., maternal consumption during pregnancy, flavors transmitted via breastmilk), then consumption in childhood may be more difficult (Raggio & Gámbaro, 2018). However, in this instance, forcing their consumption is known to be counterproductive (Raggio & Gámbaro, 2018), and a more favorable approach is to encourage consumption by creating excitement around the food and modeling enjoyable consumption (Edwards et al., 2022). Forcing consumption can also contribute to parental stress, which may hamper attempts over time and create negative perceptions and meal experiences for both parents and children (Schuster et al., 2019). Alternatively, taking approaches that do not involve force or pressure may provide protection from obesogenic exposures (e.g., food marketing) by fostering development of self-regulatory skills (Norman et al., 2018).

Breakout Box 4.1: A Parent's Perspective

As a mother whose daughter has struggled with obesity over the course of her life, I have become increasingly aware of my household's nutritional habits. I initially became concerned about my daughter's weight when she was merely 2 years old, and it seemed that her appetite was large. Having little knowledge or resources about nutrition, her weight felt unmanageable. For years, we saw specialists, ran tests, and gave countless blood samples. Eventually, I faced an extreme mental battle between continuing her extensive treatments, or simply letting her be a kid. Together, we decided that she deserved time to be a child rather than constantly being consumed by thoughts of her obesity. Looking back, I wish I would have stayed consistent with her treatments.

There have also been financial factors that have created barriers to getting my daughter the resources she needs. My husband and I work long hours and our insurance makes an insignificant dent in my daughter's medical bills; sometimes it feels as if we are in a single-income household. I have felt immense guilt for allowing my daughter to become obese, for working instead of being with her, and for not being financially able to buy healthier foods. Through all of this, my source of hope has continued to be my daughter. She is strong and resilient; she is invested in her eating habits and is stricter with herself than I am.

From the advice given to us by nutrition specialists, we have made changes in our household habits. I pack my daughter's lunches for school, we track carbohydrates and sugars, and we are particular about the menu items we choose. Although we have faced many hardships, I know that without the help we have received from professionals, we would not be on the progressive track we are today; I know that without my daughter's bravery, I could not be as positive as I am now. It is my greatest hope that my daughter will not have to face much of this once she graduates high school, and I will continue to devote myself to that effort.

—Mother of a 14-year-old daughter

The relationship between parental and child diet also extends to eating behavior. Dysregulation of eating behavior (e.g., high disinhibition) in adults has shown to influence the diets and weight of offspring (Hood et al., 2000; Jacobi et al., 2008). Specifically, maternal disinhibition (e.g., eating in response to particular stimuli, such as stress) (Hays & Roberts, 2008) is an independent predictor of daughters' weight (Cutting et al., 1999), maternal dieting is predictive of daughter dieting before age 11 (Coffman et al., 2016), and maternal emotional eating is predictive of sons' emotional eating (Jahnke & Warschburger, 2008). Increased attention has been paid to the influence of paternal eating behavior and diet, with evidence suggestive of similar effects (e.g., fathers' consumption of sweet and fat food is associated with child consumption) (Litchford et al., 2020). Additional effects are observed with family-wide habits, including cooking and consuming home meals together (van der Horst et al., 2014). This persistent and long-lasting interconnectedness between parent and child diet and eating behavior points to a critical conundrum as poor dietary patterns in the US continue: if the diets of US adults are poor, and these poor diets influence the diets of their children, how do we break the cycle?

4.4 Motivational Interviewing as an Intervention Backbone

Motivational Interviewing (MI) was originally created by William Miller and Stephen Rollnick in the 1980s as a means to help patients struggling with substance use disorders who were commonly regarded as unmotivated (Miller & Rollnick, 2023). It has been applied as an intervention strategy across a variety of behavioral domains, including those related to diet (Resnicow et al., 2015). At the heart of MI is a strong sense of mutual respect, in which a practitioner and a recipient are treated as equals with complementary expertise. From the practitioner perspective, MI is characterized by both relational and technical skills that provide a flexible yet well-defined intervention strategy. The relational skills (known as the spirit of MI) emphasize accurate empathy, honoring autonomy, collaboration, and other "soft" skills. The technical skills build upon the spirit of MI, by providing practitioners with a concrete set of tools to increase individual language in favor of changing as a means to increase and leverage intrinsic motivation to move toward behavior change (Miller & Rollnick, 2023).

As greater appreciation exists for the non-modifiable determinants of health behavior (e.g., the food environment), the field of medicine is at a crossroads: how can individuals be supported in the process of behavior change when they are faced with an ever-challenging environment that makes change exceedingly difficult? Motivational interviewing, including in the context of pediatric obesity, has been acknowledged as a key strategy, including from the American Academy of Pediatrics as part of the Clinical Practice Guideline for the Evaluation and Treatment of Children and Adolescents with Obesity (Hampl et al., 2023). With its direct emphasis on accurate empathy, MI provides a framework by which the challenges associated with non-modifiable factors and the impact these have on health and behavior can be acknowledged while still ultimately making progress toward change. This approach improves upon traditional perspectives that poor diet is secondary to a lack of motivation, but rather a feeling of ambivalence given the relative advantages and disadvantages of changing.

Motivational interviewing is commonly employed as a sole intervention, or combined with other strategies. It is flexible; as it is not itself a theory or model of behavior change, but rather a more specific way in which such frameworks can be implemented via an interventionist. It has been previously used in the context of self-determination theory (Coumans et al., 2022), the health belief model (Parwati et al., 2021), and others (Makin et al., 2021), and used alongside other approaches, such as acceptance and commitment therapy (Butryn et al., 2018), to address many health behaviors (e.g., diet, physical activity, medication adherence, and others). Indeed, combined approaches have been shown to enhance the efficacy of MI interventions (Beck et al., 2021; Moyers & Houck, 2011).

Motivational interviewing has long been considered an optimal candidate when facilitating change within families, parents, and children to improve health behavior. Such interventions have included those targeting families (O'Kane et al., 2019), children (Söderlund et al., 2009), and/or parents (Braun et al., 2023), as well as targeting various behavioral endpoints (e.g., child diet, parent diet, food environment) (Kao et al., 2023). Specifically in the area of child weight and/or obesity, a recent systematic review by Lutaud and colleagues finds that MI leads to positive behavioral and anthropometric outcomes, as well as psychological outcomes, including depression, self-efficacy, and quality of life, whereas controls experienced decreases in these outcomes (Lutaud et al., 2023). Motivational interviewing is particularly impactful when including both parents and children, though direct parental involvement may be less helpful for adolescents given a desire for more independence (Lutaud et al., 2023). Recent work has explored the development of MI-specific tools to facilitate changes in parent and child behavior, such as conversational agents that can be used to help parents navigate decisions regarding healthy food (Smriti et al., 2022).

Considering its historical use for targeting behaviors that are challenging to modify, and are not solely the result of insufficient knowledge (e.g., substance use), MI holds strong potential as a means to improve diet. Given the influence of non-modifiable factors on dietary consumption and eating behavior, but ultimately the need for some degree of individual-level change, the empathetic approach characteristic of MI can provide an optimal approach to make progress toward change while acknowledging the difficulty in doing so. In addition, given the omnipresence of many challenging factors (e.g., presence of UPF in the built food environment), facilitating the development of resilience in recipients is a potential avenue to effectively target eating behavior and ultimately diet (Heilemann et al., 2011; Lee et al., 2021).

4.5 Implications

4.5.1 Implications for Understanding Family Resilience

The influence of food manifests across all systems within the family (Henry et al., 2015). As illustrated by these systems, a key role of parents is to provide access to food (e.g., the maintenance system). Challenges (e.g., food insecurity) that can complicate this fundamental task can have profound impacts on parental stress, mental health, feeding styles, and eating behavior (Berge et al., 2020). This includes the stress of accessing food, whether or not the food accessed is considered healthy, the stress of time associated with food preparation, and whether or not it will be accepted by children. In addition to assisting parents in navigating support systems (e.g., Supplemental Nutrition Assistance Program), facilitating a shift in focus from pressuring children to eat a certain way to showing them how to eat provides an opportunity to lower stress and improve resilience.

In addition to food security status, the retail food environment and larger community- and societal-level factors to which children, adults, and families are exposed can have consequential and long-lasting effects of eating behavior, diet, and health. In the instance that food access can be augmented via navigation of support systems, parents' optimization of their own eating behavior and dietary patterns can be used to model and foster family-wide flexible rules and boundaries (e.g., the control system) (Henry et al., 2015). This is an essential element to encourage when supporting families, given parent diet and improved eating behavior can moderate response to these environments. For example, assisting parents in minimizing disinhibition and emotional eating may simultaneously help children develop positive relationships with food, and teach them to minimize use of food as a means of emotional regulation (e.g., the emotion system) (Jahnke & Warschburger, 2008). Further, the foods parents procure and prepare and the perceptions of these foods (e.g., articulating excitement regarding eating vegetables) can serve as a source of culture, optimism, and identity for families (Edwards et al., 2022). Integrating "healthy" food (e.g., fruits, vegetables) into these systems may serve as a means to ensure early and ongoing acceptance and preference among children, helping to minimize long-term reliance on more problematic foods (e.g., UPF) that ultimately contribute to obesity risk. These changes, though promising, are difficult for parents to execute, and a key component in this process is a thoughtful and empathic interventionist or clinician.

4.5.2 Implications for Practice and/or Policy

A primary and essential priority in addressing the poor dietary patterns, suboptimal eating behavior, and rate of obesity in the US is assurance that families have regular, affordable access to healthy food (Goode et al., 2023). At the forefront of this effort should include strategies to improve access to food via grocery stores and supermarkets with a variety of food options while supporting food producers by streamlining procedures and processes by which fresh food can get to consumers. Policies illustrative of this include the 2018 Farm Bill, which included approval for funds to test Produce Prescription Programs, bridging the gap between health care and food producers (Mozaffarian et al., 2019). In addition, however, policies are needed that afford families the time and mental bandwidth needed to execute the tasks needed to procure and prepare healthy food (Folta et al., 2022; Wolfson et al., 2019). These efforts should occur alongside strategies to minimize consumption of UPF, such as prohibiting the use of cartoon characters on packaging, as well as optimizing their formulation to mitigate the behavioral and health effects these foods currently appear to have (Pomeranz et al., 2023; Popkin et al., 2021).

As practitioners, utilizing approaches such as MI that place a direct emphasis on empathetic, active listening is of paramount importance. Navigating retail food environments, nutrition information, and changing diet in any capacity is exceedingly difficult, particularly when children are involved. Thus, advancing beyond strategies that center on knowledge provision is critical, and this concept is supported by existing empirical evidence (Frey et al., 2021). Motivational interviewing is a logical candidate given its purpose and original use for difficult-to-modify behaviors that are the by-product of complex exposures and experiences, and rarely secondary to insufficient knowledge (e.g., substance use disorder). Using approaches based in MI can assist practitioners in artfully and respectfully understanding exactly what behavior is occurring, why it is happening and why change is necessary, and how the change can occur. This can include connecting to community resources and support systems to ensure sufficient access to food, but can still focus on strategic conversation and problem-solving that can assist parents in changing their own diet. This includes helping connect the dots between current behavioral patterns, concerns of these patterns in the long term, and benefits of changing. Once this occurs, continued support is essential to facilitate and optimize eating behavior and food choices for parents and ultimately children.

4.6 Conclusion and Future Directions

While the retail food environment in the US needs to change, including improved access to fresh food (e.g., fruits and vegetables), it is unlikely that problematic foods (e.g., UPF) will be completely eliminated from the food landscape. Not only do these foods have the potential to modify eating behavior and health, but they are disproportionally marketed to high-risk (e.g., low-income) members of society (James et al., 2014). Thus, their behavioral effects may only serve to exacerbate those that result from similar experiences (e.g., food insecurity) (Berge et al., 2020; Goode et al., 2023). These behavioral effects may persist into childhood and/or adulthood (Yee et al., 2017), and do so independently of the effects of food insecurity (O'Connor et al., 2023).

Given the omnipresence of unhealthy foods, developing, testing, and evaluating interventions that seek to support parents in modifying their own eating behavior and food choices in order to break this cycle is critical, but per existing behavior change evidence, these interventions should not be focused solely on supplying knowledge or education. Rather, they should leverage approaches like MI that are autonomy-supportive and empathetic, but ultimately can still be used to progress toward behavior change. Indeed, MI is difficult to master and deliver in an accurate fashion, but it has a strong empirical base and is well-operationalized, meaning it can be taught, evaluated, and implemented in well-controlled and real-world settings. Conducting high-quality trials to understand the utility of MI, in order to inform the development of alternative effective interventions if necessary, is of upmost importance. However, it cannot be over-emphasized that these should occur in conjunction with approaches to improve food access and retail food environments, for example, integrating produce prescription programs and MI to simultaneously augment access to healthy food and render behavioral support to help navigate the complex dietary change and/or underlying problematic eating behavior that exists. Better yet, these should be used to bolster the development and implementation of policies to decrease the appeal of UPF to further assist in minimizing consumption.

Discussion Questions

1. How should families be encouraged to regularly consume healthy foods, while only consuming energy-dense foods (e.g., sugar-sweetened beverages) in moderation, without setting rules that are overly restrictive and contribute to disordered eating?
2. Should behavior change be supported when larger political, social, or environmental issues may be the primary drivers of suboptimal diets?
3. Should eating behavior be addressed for families struggling with food insecurity? If so, how?
4. How can the public health and healthcare community encourage use of motivational interviewing in clinical practice to assist families in change?

References

Adolph, T. E., & Tilg, H. (2024). Western diets and chronic diseases. *Nature Medicine, 30*(8), 2133–2147. https://doi.org/10.1038/s41591-024-03165-6

Beck, A. K., Baker, A. L., Carter, G., Robinson, L., McCarter, K., Wratten, C., Bauer, J., Wolfenden, L., & Britton, B. (2021). Is fidelity to a complex behaviour change intervention associated with patient outcomes? Exploring the relationship between dietitian adherence and competence and the nutritional status of intervention patients in a successful stepped-wedge randomised clinical trial of eating as treatment (EAT). *Implementation Science, 16*(1), 46. https://doi.org/10.1186/s13012-021-01118-y

Berge, J. M., Fertig, A. R., Trofholz, A., Neumark-Sztainer, D., Rogers, E., & Loth, K. (2020). Associations between parental stress, parent feeding practices, and child eating behaviors within the context of food insecurity. *Preventive Medicine Reports, 19*, 101146. https://doi.org/10.1016/j.pmedr.2020.101146

Bernard, A., Ancel, D., Neyrinck, A. M., Dastugue, A., Bindels, L. B., Delzenne, N. M., & Besnard, P. (2019). A preventive prebiotic supplementation improves the sweet taste perception in diet-induced obese mice. *Nutrients, 11*(3), Article 3. https://doi.org/10.3390/nu11030549

Blanchette, L., & Brug, J. (2005). Determinants of fruit and vegetable consumption among 6-12-year-old children and effective interventions to increase consumption. *Journal of Human Nutrition and Dietetics: The Official Journal of the British Dietetic Association, 18*(6), 431–443. https://doi.org/10.1111/j.1365-277X.2005.00648.x

Boone-Heinonen, J., Weeks, H. M., Sturza, J., Miller, A. L., Lumeng, J. C., & Bauer, K. W. (2019). Prenatal predictors of objectively-measured appetite regulation in low-income toddlers and preschool age children. *Pediatric Obesity, 14*(11), e12554. https://doi.org/10.1111/ijpo.12554

Braun, A., Portner, J., Xu, M., Weaver, L., Pratt, K., Darragh, A., & Spees, C. K. (2023). Preliminary support for the use of motivational interviewing to improve parent/adult caregiver behavior for obesity and cancer prevention. *International Journal of Environmental Research and Public Health, 20*(6), 4726. https://doi.org/10.3390/ijerph20064726

Brecic, R., Gorton, M., & Cvencek, D. (2022). Development of children's implicit and explicit attitudes toward healthy food: Personal and environmental factors. *Appetite, 176*, 106094. https://doi.org/10.1016/j.appet.2022.106094

Bryant, E. J., Rehman, J., Pepper, L. B., & Walters, E. R. (2019). Obesity and eating disturbance: The role of TFEQ restraint and disinhibition. *Current Obesity Reports, 8*(4), 363–372. https://doi.org/10.1007/s13679-019-00365-x

Butryn, M. L., Schumacher, L. M., & Forman, E. M. (2018). Alternative behavioral weight loss approaches: Acceptance and commitment therapy and motivational interviewing. In *Handbook of obesity treatment* (2nd ed., pp. 508–521). The Guilford Press.

Coffman, D. L., Balantekin, K. N., & Savage, J. S. (2016). Using propensity score methods to assess causal effects of mothers' dieting behavior on daughters' early dieting behavior. *Childhood Obesity, 12*(5), 334–340. https://doi.org/10.1089/chi.2015.0249

Contreras-Rodriguez, O., Solanas, M., & Escorihuela, R. M. (2022). Dissecting ultra-processed foods and drinks: Do they have a potential to impact the brain? *Reviews in Endocrine & Metabolic Disorders, 23*(4), 697–717. https://doi.org/10.1007/s11154-022-09711-2

Cordain, L., Eaton, S. B., Sebastian, A., Mann, N., Lindeberg, S., Watkins, B. A., O'Keefe, J. H., & Brand-Miller, J. (2005). Origins and evolution of the Western diet: Health implications for the 21st century. *The American Journal of Clinical Nutrition, 81*(2), 341–354. https://doi.org/10.1093/ajcn.81.2.341

Coumans, J. M. J., Bolman, C. A. W., Oenema, A., & Lechner, L. (2022). The effects of a web-based computer-tailored diet and physical activity intervention based on self-determination theory and motivational interviewing: A randomized controlled trial. *Internet Interventions, 28*, 100537. https://doi.org/10.1016/j.invent.2022.100537

Cutting, T. M., Fisher, J. O., Grimm-Thomas, K., & Birch, L. L. (1999). Like mother, like daughter: Familial patterns of overweight are mediated by mothers' dietary disinhibition. *The American Journal of Clinical Nutrition, 69*(4), 608–613. https://doi.org/10.1093/ajcn/69.4.608

Dai, J., Soto, M. J., Dunn, C. G., & Bleich, S. N. (2021). Trends and patterns in sugar-sweetened beverage consumption among children and adults by race and/or ethnicity, 2003-2018. *Public Health Nutrition, 24*(9), 2405–2410. https://doi.org/10.1017/S1368980021001580

Dakanalis, A., Mentzelou, M., Papadopoulou, S. K., Papandreou, D., Spanoudaki, M., Vasios, G. K., Pavlidou, E., Mantzorou, M., & Giaginis, C. (2023). The association of emotional eating with overweight/obesity, depression, anxiety/stress, and dietary patterns: A review of the current clinical evidence. *Nutrients, 15*(5), Article 5. https://doi.org/10.3390/nu15051173

De Amicis, R., Mambrini, S. P., Pellizzari, M., Foppiani, A., Bertoli, S., Battezzati, A., & Leone, A. (2022). Ultra-processed foods and obesity and adiposity parameters among children and adolescents: A systematic review. *European Journal of Nutrition, 61*(5), 2297–2311. https://doi.org/10.1007/s00394-022-02873-4

De Leon, A., Roemmich, J., & Casperson, S. (2019). Responses on the Three Factor Eating Questionnaire restraint and disinhibition scales change after a controlled energy-restricted diet (P21-002-19). *Current Developments in Nutrition, 3*, nzz041.P21-002-19. https://doi.org/10.1093/cdn/nzz041.P21-002-19

Edwards, K. L., Thomas, J. M., Higgs, S., & Blissett, J. (2022). Exposure to models' positive facial expressions whilst eating a raw vegetable increases children's acceptance and consumption of the modelled vegetable. *Appetite, 168*, 105779. https://doi.org/10.1016/j.appet.2021.105779

Folta, S. C., Anyanwu, O., Pustz, J., Oslund, J., Penkert, L. P., & Wilson, N. (2022). Food choice with economic scarcity and time abundance: A qualitative study. *Health Education & Behavior: The Official Publication of the Society for Public Health Education, 49*(1), 150–158. https://doi.org/10.1177/10901981211045926

Forestell, C. A., & Mennella, J. A. (2007). Early determinants of fruit and vegetable acceptance. *Pediatrics, 120*(6), 1247–1254. https://doi.org/10.1542/peds.2007-0858

Freedman, D. A., Bell, B. A., Clark, J. K., Sharpe, P. A., Trapl, E. S., Borawski, E. A., Pike, S. N., Rouse, C., & Sehgal, A. R. (2019). Socioecological path analytic model of diet quality among residents in two urban food deserts. *Journal of the Academy of Nutrition and Dietetics, 119*(7), 1150–1159. https://doi.org/10.1016/j.jand.2019.02.012

Frey, A. J., Lee, J., Small, J. W., Sibley, M., Owens, J. S., Skidmore, B., Johnson, L., Bradshaw, C. P., & Moyers, T. B. (2021). Mechanisms of motivational interviewing: A conceptual framework to guide practice and research. *Prevention Science, 22*(6), 689–700. https://doi.org/10.1007/s11121-020-01139-x

Goode, R. W., Godoy, S. M., Olson, K., Berg, S., Agbozo, B., Gwira, R., Xu, Y., Wolfe, H., Bhutani, J., & Alexander, R. (2023). "If I start panicking over having enough, then I start eating too much": Understanding the eating behaviors of SNAP recipients in larger bodies during COVID-19. *Eating Behaviors, 49*, 101741. https://doi.org/10.1016/j.eatbeh.2023.101741

Goswami, C., Iwasaki, Y., & Yada, T. (2018). Short-chain fatty acids suppress food intake by activating vagal afferent neurons. *The Journal of Nutritional Biochemistry, 57*, 130–135. https://doi.org/10.1016/j.jnutbio.2018.03.009

Hall, K. D., Ayuketah, A., Brychta, R., Cai, H., Cassimatis, T., Chen, K. Y., Chung, S. T., Costa, E., Courville, A., Darcey, V., Fletcher, L. A., Forde, C. G., Gharib, A. M., Guo, J., Howard, R., Joseph, P. V., McGehee, S., Ouwerkerk, R., Raisinger, K., et al. (2019). Ultra-processed diets cause excess calorie intake and weight gain: An inpatient randomized controlled trial of ad libitum food intake. *Cell Metabolism, 30*(1), 67–77.e3. https://doi.org/10.1016/j.cmet.2019.05.008

Hampl, S. E., Hassink, S. G., Skinner, A. C., Armstrong, S. C., Barlow, S. E., Bolling, C. F., Avila Edwards, K. C., Eneli, I., Hamre, R., Joseph, M. M., Lunsford, D., Mendonca, E., Michalsky, M. P., Mirza, N., Ochoa, E. R., Jr., Sharifi, M., Staiano, A. E., Weedn, A. E., Flinn, S. K., et al. (2023). Clinical practice guideline for the evaluation and treatment of children and adolescents with obesity. *Pediatrics, 151*(2), e2022060640. https://doi.org/10.1542/peds.2022-060640

Hays, N. P., & Roberts, S. B. (2008). Aspects of eating behaviors "disinhibition" and "restraint" are related to weight gain and BMI in women. *Obesity, 16*(1), 52–58. https://doi.org/10.1038/oby.2007.12

Heilemann, M. V., Pieters, H. C., Kehoe, P., & Yang, Q. (2011). Schema therapy, motivational interviewing, and collaborative-mapping as treatment for depression among low income, second generation Latinas. *Journal of Behavior Therapy and Experimental Psychiatry, 42*(4), 473–480. https://doi.org/10.1016/j.jbtep.2011.05.001

Henry, C. S., Sheffield Morris, A., & Harrist, A. W. (2015). Family resilience: Moving into the third wave. *Family Relations, 64*(1), 22–43. https://doi.org/10.1111/fare.12106

Hetherington, M. M., Schwartz, C., Madrelle, J., Croden, F., Nekitsing, C., Vereijken, C. M. J. L., & Weenen, H. (2015). A step-by-step introduction to vegetables at the beginning of complementary feeding. The effects of early and repeated exposure. *Appetite, 84*, 280–290. https://doi.org/10.1016/j.appet.2014.10.014

Hood, M. Y., Moore, L. L., Sundarajan-Ramamurti, A., Singer, M., Cupples, L. A., & Ellison, R. C. (2000). Parental eating attitudes and the development of obesity in children. The Framingham Children's Study. *International Journal of Obesity, 24*(10), Article 10. https://doi.org/10.1038/sj.ijo.0801396

Hung, L.-S., Tidwell, D. K., Hall, M. E., Lee, M. L., Briley, C. A., & Hunt, B. P. (2015). A meta-analysis of school-based obesity prevention programs demonstrates limited efficacy of decreasing childhood obesity. *Nutrition Research, 35*(3), 229–240. https://doi.org/10.1016/j.nutres.2015.01.002

Hunot, C., Fildes, A., Croker, H., Llewellyn, C. H., Wardle, J., & Beeken, R. J. (2016). Appetitive traits and relationships with BMI in adults: Development of the adult eating behaviour questionnaire. *Appetite, 105*, 356–363. https://doi.org/10.1016/j.appet.2016.05.024

Jacobi, C., Schmitz, G., & Agras, W. S. (2008). Interactions between disturbed eating and weight in children and their mothers. *Journal of Developmental and Behavioral Pediatrics, 29*(5), 360–366. https://doi.org/10.1097/DBP.0b013e31817dbd7d

Jahnke, D. L., & Warschburger, P. A. (2008). Familial transmission of eating behaviors in preschool-aged children. *Obesity, 16*(8), 1821–1825. https://doi.org/10.1038/oby.2008.255

James, P., Arcaya, M. C., Parker, D. M., & Tucker-Seeley, R. (2014). Do minority and poor neighborhoods have higher access to fast-food restaurants in the United States? *Health & Place, 29*, 10–17. https://doi.org/10.1016/j.healthplace.2014.04.011

Järvelä-Reijonen, E., Karhunen, L., Sairanen, E., Muotka, J., Lindroos, S., Laitinen, J., Puttonen, S., Peuhkuri, K., Hallikainen, M., Pihlajamäki, J., Korpela, R., Ermes, M., Lappalainen, R., & Kolehmainen, M. (2018). The effects of acceptance and commitment therapy on eating behavior and diet delivered through face-to-face contact and a mobile app: A randomized controlled trial. *The International Journal of Behavioral Nutrition and Physical Activity, 15*(1), 22. https://doi.org/10.1186/s12966-018-0654-8

Johnson, F., Pratt, M., & Wardle, J. (2012). Dietary restraint and self-regulation in eating behavior. *International Journal of Obesity, 36*(5), 665–674. https://doi.org/10.1038/ijo.2011.156

Juul, F., Parekh, N., Martinez-Steele, E., Monteiro, C. A., & Chang, V. W. (2022). Ultra-processed food consumption among US adults from 2001 to 2018. *The American Journal of Clinical Nutrition, 115*(1), 211–221. https://doi.org/10.1093/ajcn/nqab305

Kaczmarczyk, M. M., Miller, M. J., & Freund, G. G. (2012). The health benefits of dietary fiber: Beyond the usual suspects of type 2 diabetes, cardiovascular disease and colon cancer. *Metabolism, 61*(8), 1058–1066. https://doi.org/10.1016/j.metabol.2012.01.017

Kao, T.-S. A., Ling, J., Vu, C., Hawn, R., & Christodoulos, H. (2023). Motivational interviewing in pediatric obesity: A meta-analysis of the effects on behavioral outcomes. *Annals of Behavioral Medicine, 57*(8), 605–619. https://doi.org/10.1093/abm/kaad006

Kimmons, J., Gillespie, C., Seymour, J., Serdula, M., & Blanck, H. M. (2009). Fruit and vegetable intake among adolescents and adults in the United States: Percentage meeting individualized recommendations. *The Medscape Journal of Medicine, 11*(1), 26.

Koh, A., Vadder, F. D., Kovatcheva-Datchary, P., & Bäckhed, F. (2016). From dietary fiber to host physiology: Short-chain fatty acids as key bacterial metabolites. *Cell, 165*(6), 1332–1345. https://doi.org/10.1016/j.cell.2016.05.041

Konttinen, H., van Strien, T., Männistö, S., Jousilahti, P., & Haukkala, A. (2019). Depression, emotional eating and long-term weight changes: A population-based prospective study. *The International Journal of Behavioral Nutrition and Physical Activity, 16*, 28. https://doi.org/10.1186/s12966-019-0791-8

Lee, J. A., Heberlein, E., Pyle, E., Caughlan, T., Rahaman, D., Sabin, M., & Kaar, J. L. (2021). Evaluation of a resiliency focused health coaching intervention for middle school students: Building resilience for healthy kids program. *American Journal of Health Promotion, 35*(3), 344–351. https://doi.org/10.1177/0890117120959152

Lee, S. H. (2022). Adults meeting fruit and vegetable intake recommendations—United States, 2019. *MMWR. Morbidity and Mortality Weekly Report, 71*. https://doi.org/10.15585/mmwr.mm7101a1

Leung, C. W., Fulay, A. P., Parnarouskis, L., Martinez-Steele, E., Gearhardt, A. N., & Wolfson, J. A. (2022). Food insecurity and ultra-processed food consumption: The modifying role of participation in the Supplemental Nutrition Assistance Program (SNAP). *The American Journal of Clinical Nutrition, 116*(1), 197–205. https://doi.org/10.1093/ajcn/nqac049

Litchford, A., Savoie Roskos, M. R., & Wengreen, H. (2020). Influence of fathers on the feeding practices and behaviors of children: A systematic review. *Appetite, 147*, 104558. https://doi.org/10.1016/j.appet.2019.104558

Liu, J., Micha, R., Li, Y., & Mozaffarian, D. (2021a). Trends in food sources and diet quality among US children and adults, 2003-2018. *JAMA Network Open, 4*(4), e215262. https://doi.org/10.1001/jamanetworkopen.2021.5262

Liu, X., Li, X., Xia, B., Jin, X., Zou, Q., Zeng, Z., Zhao, W., Yan, S., Li, L., Yuan, S., Zhao, S., Dai, X., Yin, F., Cadenas, E., Liu, R. H., Zhao, B., Hou, M., Liu, Z., & Liu, X. (2021b). High-fiber diet mitigates maternal obesity-induced cognitive and social dysfunction in the offspring via gut-brain axis. *Cell Metabolism, 33*(5), 923–938.e6. https://doi.org/10.1016/j.cmet.2021.02.002

Lopez, N. V., Schembre, S., Belcher, B. R., O'Connor, S., Maher, J. P., Arbel, R., Margolin, G., & Dunton, G. F. (2018). Parenting styles, food-related parenting practices, and children's healthy eating: A mediation analysis to examine relationships between parenting and child diet. *Appetite, 128*, 205–213. https://doi.org/10.1016/j.appet.2018.06.021

Lorts, C., Tasevska, N., Adams, M. A., Yedidia, M. J., Tulloch, D., Hooker, S. P., & Ohri-Vachaspati, P. (2019). Participation in the Supplemental Nutrition Assistance Program and dietary behaviors: Role of community food environment. *Journal of the Academy of Nutrition and Dietetics, 119*(6), 934–943.e2. https://doi.org/10.1016/j.jand.2018.11.021

Lutaud, R., Mitilian, E., Forte, J., Gentile, G., Reynaud, R., Truffet, C., & Bellanger, T. (2023). Motivational interviewing for the management of child and adolescent obesity: A systematic literature review. *BJGP Open*. https://doi.org/10.3399/BJGPO.2022.0145

Makin, H., Chisholm, A., Fallon, V., & Goodwin, L. (2021). Use of motivational interviewing in behavioural interventions among adults with obesity: A systematic review and meta-analysis. *Clinical Obesity, 11*(4), e12457. https://doi.org/10.1111/cob.12457

Marijn Stok, F., Renner, B., Allan, J., Boeing, H., Ensenauer, R., Issanchou, S., Kiesswetter, E., Lien, N., Mazzocchi, M., Monsivais, P., Stelmach-Mardas, M., Volkert, D., & Hoffmann, S. (2018). Dietary behavior: An interdisciplinary conceptual analysis and taxonomy. *Frontiers in Psychology, 9*. https://doi.org/10.3389/fpsyg.2018.01689

McLeroy, K. R., Bibeau, D., Steckler, A., & Glanz, K. (1988). An ecological perspective on health promotion programs. *Health Education Quarterly, 15*(4), 351–377. https://doi.org/10.1177/109019818801500401

Medawar, E., Beyer, F., Thieleking, R., Haange, S.-B., Rolle-Kampczyk, U., Reinicke, M., Chakaroun, R., von Bergen, M., Stumvoll, M., Villringer, A., & Witte, A. V. (2024). Prebiotic diet changes neural correlates of food decision-making in overweight adults: A randomised controlled within-subject cross-over trial. *Gut, 73*(2), 298–310. https://doi.org/10.1136/gutjnl-2023-330365

Medawar, E., Haange, S.-B., Rolle-Kampczyk, U., Engelmann, B., Dietrich, A., Thieleking, R., Wiegank, C., Fries, C., Horstmann, A., Villringer, A., von Bergen, M., Fenske, W., & Veronica Witte, A. (2021). Gut microbiota link dietary fiber intake and short-chain fatty acid metabolism with eating behavior. *Translational Psychiatry, 11*(1), Article 1. https://doi.org/10.1038/s41398-021-01620-3

Mennella, J. A., Daniels, L. M., & Reiter, A. R. (2017). Learning to like vegetables during breastfeeding: A randomized clinical trial of lactating mothers and infants. *The American Journal of Clinical Nutrition, 106*(1), 67–76. https://doi.org/10.3945/ajcn.116.143982

Miller, W. R., & Rollnick, S. (2023). *Motivational interviewing: Helping people change and grow* (4th ed.). The Guilford Press.

Miyake, K., Horiuchi, S., Shinohara, R., Kushima, M., Otawa, S., Yui, H., Akiyama, Y., Ooka, T., Kojima, R., Yokomichi, H., Mochizuki, K., Yamagata, Z., & Japan Environment Children's Study Group. (2023). Maternal dietary fiber intake during pregnancy and child development: The Japan Environment and Children's Study. *Frontiers in Nutrition, 10*, 1203669. https://doi.org/10.3389/fnut.2023.1203669

Monteban, M. F., Bess, K. D., Walsh, C. C., Baily, H., Flocke, S. A., Borawski, E. A., & Freedman, D. A. (2018). People and places shaping food procurement among recipients of Supplemental Nutrition Assistance Program (SNAP). *Health & Place, 53*, 155–163. https://doi.org/10.1016/j.healthplace.2018.08.003

Monteiro, C. A., Cannon, G., Levy, R., Moubarac, J.-C., Jaime, P., Martins, A. P., Canella, D., Louzada, M., & Parra, D. (2016). NOVA. The star shines bright. *World Nutrition, 7*(1–3), Article 1–3.

Moore, L. L., Nguyen, U. S., Rothman, K. J., Cupples, L. A., & Ellison, R. C. (1995). Preschool physical activity level and change in body fatness in young children. The Framingham Children's Study. *American Journal of Epidemiology, 142*(9), 982–988. https://doi.org/10.1093/oxfordjournals.aje.a117747

Morze, J., Danielewicz, A., Hoffmann, G., & Schwingshackl, L. (2020). Diet quality as assessed by the Healthy Eating Index, Alternate Healthy Eating Index, Dietary Approaches to Stop Hypertension Score, and health outcomes: A second update of a systematic review and meta-analysis of cohort studies. *Journal of the Academy of Nutrition and Dietetics, 120*(12), 1998-2031.e15. https://doi.org/10.1016/j.jand.2020.08.076

Moyers, T. B., & Houck, J. (2011). Combining motivational interviewing with cognitive-behavioral treatments for substance abuse: Lessons from the COMBINE research project. *Cognitive and Behavioral Practice, 18*(1), 38–45. https://doi.org/10.1016/j.cbpra.2009.09.005

Mozaffarian, D., Griffin, T., & Mande, J. (2019). The 2018 Farm Bill—Implications and opportunities for public health. *JAMA, 321*(9), 835–836. https://doi.org/10.1001/jama.2019.0317

Neumann, N. J., & Fasshauer, M. (2022). Added flavors: Potential contributors to body weight gain and obesity? *BMC Medicine, 20*(1), 417. https://doi.org/10.1186/s12916-022-02619-3

Norman, Å., Nyberg, G., & Berlin, A. (2019). School-based obesity prevention for busy low-income families—Organisational and personal barriers and facilitators to implementation. *PLoS One, 14*(11), e0224512. https://doi.org/10.1371/journal.pone.0224512

Norman, J., Kelly, B., McMahon, A.-T., Boyland, E., Baur, L. A., Chapman, K., King, L., Hughes, C., & Bauman, A. (2018). Children's self-regulation of eating provides no defense against television and online food marketing. *Appetite, 125*, 438–444. https://doi.org/10.1016/j.appet.2018.02.026

O'Connor, S. M., Zickgraf, H. F., Hazzard, V. M., Haller, L. L., & Wildes, J. E. (2023). Exploring differences in disordered eating and related appetitive traits among women based on childhood and current food security status. *Eating Behaviors, 49*, 101729. https://doi.org/10.1016/j.eatbeh.2023.101729

O'Kane, C., Irwin, J. D., Morrow, D., Tang, L., Wong, S., Buchholz, A. C., Ma, D. W. L., & Haines, J. (2019). Motivational interviewing with families in the home environment. *Patient Education and Counseling, 102*(11), 2073–2080. https://doi.org/10.1016/j.pec.2019.06.002

Oliver, A., Chase, A. B., Weihe, C., Orchanian, S. B., Riedel, S. F., Hendrickson, C. L., Lay, M., Sewall, J. M., Martiny, J. B. H., & Whiteson, K. (2021). High-fiber, whole-food dietary intervention alters the human gut microbiome but not fecal short-chain fatty acids. *mSystems, 6*(2). https://doi.org/10.1128/msystems.00115-21

Papini, N. M., Foster, R. N. S., Lopez, N. V., Ptomey, L. T., Herrmann, S. D., & Donnelly, J. E. (2022). Examination of three-factor eating questionnaire subscale scores on weight loss and weight loss maintenance in a clinical intervention. *BMC Psychology, 10*(1), 101. https://doi.org/10.1186/s40359-022-00806-8

Parwati, N. M., Bakta, I. M., Januraga, P. P., & Wirawan, I. M. A. (2021). A Health Belief Model-based Motivational Interviewing for medication adherence and treatment success in pulmonary tuberculosis patients. *International Journal of Environmental Research and Public Health, 18*(24), Article 24. https://doi.org/10.3390/ijerph182413238

Pearson, N., Biddle, S. J. H., & Gorely, T. (2009). Family correlates of fruit and vegetable consumption in children and adolescents: A systematic review. *Public Health Nutrition, 12*(2), 267–283. https://doi.org/10.1017/S1368980008002589

Polivy, J., Herman, C. P., & Mills, J. S. (2020). What is restrained eating and how do we identify it? *Appetite, 155*, 104820. https://doi.org/10.1016/j.appet.2020.104820

Pomeranz, J. L., Mande, J. R., & Mozaffarian, D. (2023). U.S. policies addressing ultraprocessed foods, 1980–2022. *American Journal of Preventive Medicine, 65*(6), 1134–1141. https://doi.org/10.1016/j.amepre.2023.07.006

Popkin, B. M., Barquera, S., Corvalan, C., Hofman, K. J., Monteiro, C., Ng, S. W., Swart, E. C., & Taillie, L. S. (2021). Toward unified and impactful policies for reducing ultraprocessed food consumption and promoting healthier eating globally. *The Lancet. Diabetes & Endocrinology, 9*(7), 462–470. https://doi.org/10.1016/S2213-8587(21)00078-4

Raggio, L., & Gámbaro, A. (2018). Study of the reasons for the consumption of each type of vegetable within a population of school-aged children. *BMC Public Health, 18*, 1163. https://doi.org/10.1186/s12889-018-6067-4

Ravikumar, D., Spyreli, E., Woodside, J., McKinley, M., & Kelly, C. (2022). Parental perceptions of the food environment and their influence on food decisions among low-income families: A rapid review of qualitative evidence. *BMC Public Health, 22*(1), 9. https://doi.org/10.1186/s12889-021-12414-z

Resnicow, K., McMaster, F., Bocian, A., Harris, D., Zhou, Y., Snetselaar, L., Schwartz, R., Myers, E., Gotlieb, J., Foster, J., Hollinger, D., Smith, K., Woolford, S., Mueller, D., & Wasserman, R. C. (2015). Motivational interviewing and dietary counseling for obesity in primary care: An RCT. *Pediatrics, 135*(4), 649–657. https://doi.org/10.1542/peds.2014-1880

Saltzman, J. A., Liechty, J. M., Bost, K. K., & Fiese, B. H. (2016). Parent binge eating and restrictive feeding practices: Indirect effects of parent's responses to child's negative emotion. *Eating Behaviors, 21*, 150–154. https://doi.org/10.1016/j.eatbeh.2016.02.001

Satia, J. A., Kristal, A. R., Curry, S., & Trudeau, E. (2001). Motivations for healthful dietary change. *Public Health Nutrition, 4*(5), 953–959. https://doi.org/10.1079/phn2001157

Scaglioni, S., De Cosmi, V., Ciappolino, V., Parazzini, F., Brambilla, P., & Agostoni, C. (2018). Factors influencing children's eating behaviours. *Nutrients, 10*(6), Article 6. https://doi.org/10.3390/nu10060706

Schuster, R. C., Szpak, M., Klein, E., Sklar, K., & Dickin, K. L. (2019). "I try, I do": Child feeding practices of motivated, low-income parents reflect trade-offs between psychosocial and nutrition goals. *Appetite, 136*, 114–123. https://doi.org/10.1016/j.appet.2019.01.005

Silva, Y. P., Bernardi, A., & Frozza, R. L. (2020). The role of short-chain fatty acids from gut microbiota in gut-brain communication. *Frontiers in Endocrinology, 11*. https://doi.org/10.3389/fendo.2020.00025

Smriti, D., Kao, T.-S. A., Rathod, R., Shin, J. Y., Peng, W., Williams, J., Mujib, M. I., Colosimo, M., & Huh-Yoo, J. (2022). Motivational Interviewing conversational agent for parents as proxies for their children in healthy eating: Development and user testing. *JMIR Human Factors, 9*(4), e38908. https://doi.org/10.2196/38908

Sobol-Goldberg, S., Rabinowitz, J., & Gross, R. (2013). School-based obesity prevention programs: A meta-analysis of randomized controlled trials. *Obesity, 21*(12), 2422–2428. https://doi.org/10.1002/oby.20515

Söderlund, L. L., Nordqvist, C., Angbratt, M., & Nilsen, P. (2009). Applying motivational interviewing to counselling overweight and obese children. *Health Education Research, 24*(3), 442–449. https://doi.org/10.1093/her/cyn039

Spahn, J. M., Callahan, E. H., Spill, M. K., Wong, Y. P., Benjamin-Neelon, S. E., Birch, L., Black, M. M., Cook, J. T., Faith, M. S., Mennella, J. A., & Casavale, K. O. (2019). Influence of maternal diet on flavor transfer to amniotic fluid and breast milk and children's responses: A systematic review. *The American Journal of Clinical Nutrition, 109*, 1003S–1026S. https://doi.org/10.1093/ajcn/nqy240

Spinelli, S., & Monteleone, E. (2021). Food preferences and obesity. *Endocrinology and Metabolism, 36*(2), 209–219. https://doi.org/10.3803/EnM.2021.105

Stunkard, A. J., & Messick, S. (1985). The three-factor eating questionnaire to measure dietary restraint, disinhibition and hunger. *Journal of Psychosomatic Research, 29*(1), 71–83. https://doi.org/10.1016/0022-3999(85)90010-8

Thomas, J. G., Doshi, S., Crosby, R. D., & Lowe, M. R. (2011). Ecological momentary assessment of obesogenic eating behavior: Combining person-specific and environmental predictors. *Obesity, 19*(8), 1574–1579. https://doi.org/10.1038/oby.2010.335

Tseng, M., Grigsby, C. J., Austin, A., Amin, S., & Nazmi, A. (2022). Sensory-related industrial additives in the US packaged food supply. *Frontiers in Nutrition, 8*. https://doi.org/10.3389/fnut.2021.762814

van der Horst, K., Ferrage, A., & Rytz, A. (2014). Involving children in meal preparation. Effects on food intake. *Appetite, 79*, 18–24. https://doi.org/10.1016/j.appet.2014.03.030

van Strien, T. (2018). Causes of emotional eating and matched treatment of obesity. *Current Diabetes Reports, 18*(6), 35. https://doi.org/10.1007/s11892-018-1000-x

van Strien, T., Frijters, J. E. R., Bergers, G. P. A., & Defares, P. B. (1986). The Dutch Eating Behavior Questionnaire (DEBQ) for assessment of restrained, emotional, and external eating behavior. *International Journal of Eating Disorders, 5*(2), 295–315. https://doi.org/10.1002/1098-108X(198602)5:2<295::AID-EAT2260050209>3.0.CO;2-T

Vaughn, A. E., Martin, C. L., & Ward, D. S. (2018). What matters most—What parents model or what parents eat? *Appetite, 126*, 102–107. https://doi.org/10.1016/j.appet.2018.03.025

Vidal, L., Brunet, G., Bove, I., Girona, A., Fuletti, D., & Ares, G. (2021). Parents' mental associations with ultra-processed products for their infant children: Insights to improve complementary feeding practices. *Food Quality and Preference, 94*, 104335. https://doi.org/10.1016/j.foodqual.2021.104335

Wang, D. D., Li, Y., Bhupathiraju, S. N., Rosner, B. A., Sun, Q., Giovannucci, E. L., Rimm, E. B., Manson, J. E., Willett, W. C., Stampfer, M. J., & Hu, F. B. (2021a). Fruit and vegetable intake and mortality: Results from 2 prospective cohort studies of US men and women and a meta-analysis of 26 cohort studies. *Circulation, 143*(17), 1642–1654. https://doi.org/10.1161/CIRCULATIONAHA.120.048996

Wang, L., Martínez Steele, E., Du, M., Pomeranz, J. L., O'Connor, L. E., Herrick, K. A., Luo, H., Zhang, X., Mozaffarian, D., & Zhang, F. F. (2021b). Trends in consumption of ultraprocessed foods among US youths aged 2-19 years, 1999-2018. *JAMA, 326*(6), 519–530. https://doi.org/10.1001/jama.2021.10238

Wolfson, J. A., Ramsing, R., Richardson, C. R., & Palmer, A. (2019). Barriers to healthy food access: Associations with household income and cooking behavior. *Preventive Medicine Reports, 13*, 298–305. https://doi.org/10.1016/j.pmedr.2019.01.023

Yee, A. Z. H., Lwin, M. O., & Ho, S. S. (2017). The influence of parental practices on child promotive and preventive food consumption behaviors: A systematic review and meta-analysis. *International Journal of Behavioral Nutrition and Physical Activity, 14*(1), 47. https://doi.org/10.1186/s12966-017-0501-3

Chapter 5
Disordered Eating and Resilience in Trans and Gender Diverse Populations

Bek Urban, Sebastian M. Barr, and Douglas Knutson

Scholars suggest that studies of family resilience have moved into a third wave marked by a more complex and systems-oriented understanding of resilience that shifts well beyond individual-focused models (Henry et al., 2015). New ways of approaching resilience take into account sociocultural contexts, interpersonal dynamics, and collective stress management. However, research on marginalized groups remains damage-centered and individual-focused. In other words, when conceptualizing or framing marginalized communities, scholars, practitioners, and society more broadly tend to focus on negative outcomes (e.g., distress, poor health) and they frame distressed individuals as both the problem and solution to their own suffering. For example, disordered eating and body image concerns in trans and nonbinary (TNB) people are generally attributed to the difficulties of being TNB and the responsibility for stemming the tide of disordered eating and negative body image is placed squarely on the shoulders of TNB people.

Third wave models of family resilience challenge established approaches to distress and coping in marginalized populations, such as TNB people. Counter to current trends, third wave models call scholars and practitioners to recognize that disordered eating and body image concerns take shape in a much broader sociocultural context. For example, they are influenced by sociocultural context and interpersonal dynamics. Building on this third wave model of resilience, researchers have started to identify ways that compound trauma that originates in society plays a major role in producing distress, dysfunction, disordered eating, and body image

B. Urban (✉) · D. Knutson
School of Community Health Sciences, Counseling and Counseling Psychology, Oklahoma State University, Stillwater, OK, USA
e-mail: rebekah.e.urban@okstate.edu

S. M. Barr
Private Practice, MA, USA

G. Welch et al. (eds.), *Stress, Resilience, and Healthy Relationships with Food and Family*, Emerging Issues in Family and Individual Resilience,
https://doi.org/10.1007/978-3-031-98937-7_5

concerns. In other words, the responsibility for distress and maladaptive coping behaviors rests with society itself.

Writers heralding the third wave of family resilience science also remind scholars to investigate, emphasize, and better understand the role of resilience and resistance in the lives of TNB people. Researchers, scholars, and the general public are invited to simultaneously acknowledge the suffering faced by TNB people while also embracing the powerful resilience strategies TNB people have developed to survive and ultimately thrive in oppressive societies. If scholars and practitioners are to fully understand disordered eating, body image concerns, and other negative experiences reported by TNB people, they must adopt a more expansive model, one guided by the third wave of family resilience.

5.1 Literature Review

Most research with TNB people, including studies that investigate disordered eating and body image, has been characterized as damage-centered and individual-focused. That is, scholars tend to focus on the negative and harmful outcomes faced by members of the TNB community and they center both the problems and solutions in individual TNB people. However, eating disorder and body image treatments and interventions that are based on damage-centered and individual-focused assumptions fail to account for critical systems-level dynamics and sociocultural contexts. For example, they fail to take into account the toxicity of discriminatory attitudes among cisgender people and the empowering effect of community connections among TNB people.

Researchers have pointed out that this problem focus negatively impacts TNB people when, for example, it leads to the assumption that TNB people are inherently disordered because of the experiences of distress that are commonly reported by TNB people (Levitt et al., 2023). In response to the dominant focus on distress, scholars have started to shift to researching phenomena such as trans empowerment, liberation, and gender euphoria. However, due to oppressive social systems in which TNB people exist, it is nearly impossible to focus solely on either harm or beauty. In this chapter, we will focus on both with an emphasis on the strengths and resilience exhibited by TNB people. We encourage readers to keep in mind the incredible tenacity and bravery within TNB communities.

For example, Zimman (2019) writes about the ways in which trans self-determination related to gender expression is liberatory. Liberation, however, generally occurs and is emphasized "in the face of brutality and trauma" (p.172). In other words, investigations of TNB strength and resilience must contain a dual awareness of the roles of both liberation *and* trauma, of harm *and* beauty. In this chapter, we acknowledge the challenges and risks faced by many TNB individuals especially related to disordered eating and body image, but we also work to push back against assumptions that harm within TNB communities is tied to being trans itself. Instead, we ground our discussion in the sociocultural context of oppression, stigma, and trauma that TNB people experience on a daily basis. It is in this reality that harm is enacted against TNB individuals, and in which trans individuals find joy, euphoria, resilience, and resistance.

5.1.1 Trans and Nonbinary People in Sociocultural Contexts

TNB people experience structural and enacted stigma from multiple sources at multiple ecological levels (e.g., structural and interpersonal). Examples of such stigma include signals of hostile sociocultural climates, experiences of bias (e.g., rejection, discrimination, alienation), violence and threats of violence, and non-affirmation and invalidation of their gender and trans identities. For many if not most TNB people, direct (in which they are the target) and indirect (in which they witness harm to others) experiences of identity-based harm occur daily across different sectors/spheres of their lives, and the accumulation of these injuries can be a significant psychological burden. Although sometimes enacted and structural stigma takes the form of severe and externally visible assault, such as physical violence or being fired, these experiences more often fall in the category of what gender studies professor Dr. Hil Malatino describes as "trans traumas of the mundane" (2022, p. 6). These are commonplace experiences of identity-based harm, related to the concept of microaggressions, which still have the power to wear down their targets and motivate the reorganization of behaviors such as ways of engaging with the self and/or others in an effort to maintain psychological and/or physical safety. Psychologist and trauma expert Dr. Laura Brown uses the metaphor of acid rain on stone to emphasize the cumulative impacts and risks of these ordinary, compounding traumas:

> Each drop by itself does little damage and may in fact etch the stone in such a way as to make it more beautiful. Thus, in some way the experience of daily microaggressions may evoke resilient coping responses. Yet each drop of emotion acid creates just enough damage to render the next drop more damaging. At times the dilution of the acid is such that the particular microaggression is barely perceived; at other times its sting is more apparent… Over time a fissure develops in the form of an emotional vulnerability that is invisible so long as certain aspects of the biopsychosocial and spiritual environment remain steady or supportive. (Brown, 2008, p. 104)

Brown (2008) continues this metaphor, writing that symptoms or signs of traumatization present "when enough acid has fallen" or when the environment fails to be an adequate source of support and resilience (p. 104). Relevant to this concept are the ways in which other stigmatized and oppressed identities, experiences, and backgrounds further shape TNB people's sociocultural and interpersonal contexts—extending Brown's metaphor, these intersecting oppressions may detract from the supportive environment needed to prevent the fissure from developing into something more damaging. Although historically, clinical and research work in trans mental health has taken a "single axis" approach, treating trans people as monolith, the reality is that a person's experience of their gender, gendered oppression, trans-related oppression, and the celebratory and resilient facets of transness are all impacted by their race and ethnicity, dis/ability status, class background, gender identity, gender presentation, and so on (Bowleg et al., 2023; Chang & Singh, 2016; Wesp et al., 2019).

TNB people with intersecting marginalized identities likely experience stigma due to their transness, their other identities, and the relationship between those identities (Ching et al., 2018). For example, trans women of color tend to attribute experiences of discrimination to bias related to them being both trans women and members of minoritized racial groups (Wesson et al., 2021), and among a sample of Black LGBQ people, day-to-day negative experiences related to intersectional identities lead to more identity conflict, negative affect, and negative rumination than negative experiences attributed to a single axis of their identities (Jackson et al., 2020). Similarly, Maroney and Horne (2022) noted that for autistic trans and/or nonbinary people, daily navigation of the world involves a "complex set of intersectional processes," such that structural ableism was nearly impossible to disentangle from the structural cissexism and heterosexism in their lives. Importantly, intersectional experiences can also be positive and important sources of resilience, coping, and healing (Bryant-Davis, 2019; Jackson et al., 2020), which we will return to later in the chapter.

In terms of understanding the relationships between the ubiquitous identity-based harm (both single-axis and intersectional), scholars focusing on TNB people's lives and mental health (many of them, notably members of the TNB community themselves) have utilized a number of helpful models for framing these realities. The minority stress and resilience model emphasizes the relationship among external stressors, internal stressors, and negative health outcomes, with community-driven adaptations recently focusing more heavily on sources of resilience that can disrupt these relationships (Matsuno & Israel, 2018; Tan et al., 2019). The ecological model emphasizes the multiple systems in which bias is enacted and experienced: society, community, organizations, interpersonal relationships, and within the person themself (Puckett, 2019; Puckett et al., 2022), and is related to work on biological stress and allostatic load, which has found correlations between hostile geopolitical environments and markers of biological stress in trans men (DuBois & Juster, 2022).

We will be focusing on the trauma framework scholars and community members have put forth, as we find feminist trauma theory to be particularly helpful in understanding the etiology and roles of disordered eating behavior within these communities. In this framework, the harm identified within the gender minority stress model as distal stressors (e.g., anti-transgender bias events and non-affirmation) *and* the more structural and systemic harms captured by elements of the ecological model are understood as potentially traumatic experiences. The negative outcomes associated with these experiences (e.g., depressive symptoms, suicidality, substance use, anxiety, somatic concerns) are then conceptualized to be symptoms of complex traumatic stress (Barr, 2018; Richmond et al., 2012).

5.1.2 A Trauma Framework

Drawing from work on racial trauma, psychologists have argued that anti-transgender bias events, non-affirmation, and structural stigma constitute forms of violence that can operate as severe threats to psychological and social sense of self as well as threats to physical safety/needs (Barr et al., 2021; Colson et al., 2023; Richmond et al., 2017) particularly when these experiences accumulate as they commonly do. The chronic and often interpersonal and/or seemingly inescapable nature of this kind of trauma exposure (i.e., complex trauma) can have profound impacts on individuals' emotional experiences and capacities, self-perception, and relationships (Briere & Spinazzola, 2005; Herman, 1992). This is largely because victims develop ways of understanding themselves, others, and the world that attempt to rebuild a sense of safety, security, and control—or that otherwise allow them to make sense of the chronic harm they've experienced (Root, 1992).

These responses can be maladaptive outside of these traumatic contexts and/or cause harm to the individual or the people around them, and thus might be identified by clinicians as pathological traumatic stress symptoms (Herman, 2015), but it is critical to understand that each behavior likely developed to serve a purpose related to the trauma. For example, complex trauma survivors often develop poor self-worth and struggle with deep-seated feelings of shame. These might have developed unconsciously to aid them in understanding how someone they care about or depend on (e.g., a parent or an institution in which they're embedded) could be so harmful to them. Dissociation often develops as a protective mechanism against the pain of difficult external and internal experiences.

As we will expand upon, disordered eating and other patterns associated with eating disorders may be a way to disconnect from one's body and either preemptively numb or momentarily relieve strong, unwanted feelings. Other common pieces of complex traumatic stress include emotion regulation difficulties, avoidance, relational turbulence, and self-harm. Research has demonstrated that among TNB people, non-affirmation, discrimination, and other bias experiences are associated with increased PTSD symptom severity, and that this relationship is also related to identity-based shame, lending support for the complex trauma framework (Barr et al., 2021; Reisner et al., 2016). Further, PTSD prevalence appears to be very high in trans and nonbinary communities—studies have found rates near 45% (Barr et al., 2021; Reisner et al., 2016).

5.1.2.1 Pressure to Conform

Additionally, it is critical to understand how oppressive sociocultural contexts also shape TNB people's relationships with their bodies. Dominant standards of feminine beauty and acceptable appearance center or hyperfocus on thin, white, nondisabled, cisgender women. Masculine appearance standards may allow for more flexibility related to acceptable body size, but still place heavy emphasis on masculinity being synonymous with muscular, fit, white, nondisabled, cisgender men. Emphasis on these narrow definitions simultaneously excludes individuals who do not neatly fit into such categories while necessitating never-ending attempts to meet unattainable standards. Although these constructs are often discussed as beauty ideals or appearance aspirations, these standards must be understood as more than aspirational beauty ideals that people willingly strive for.

Pressure to attain appearance standards negatively impacts all people and exerts control over the bodies of those with less social capital. To TNB individuals, however, these standards also represent social hegemony that is completely inaccessible to individuals who are not and *cannot* be thin, white, nondisabled, and cisgender (Deliovsky, 2008). The widespread social and economic barriers trans individuals face is well documented and has tremendous impacts on TNB people's ability to more closely align with these standards (Burnes et al., 2010). When TNB individuals desire gender affirming medical care, they often find that it is costly, is poorly covered by insurance, may require trans individuals to "prove" their transness and distress to be covered by insurance, and is often restricted to TNB individuals whose bodies are below certain body mass indexes set by doctors. These barriers preclude many trans persons who desire gender affirming medical care from accessing it, which may also limit one's ability to align their gender presentation with their ideal presentation.

Although TNB individuals may engage in "everyday resistance" (GagnÉ & Tewksbury, 1998) against conformity to standards of cisnormative femininity or masculinity, potential safety and social capital that is accessible through investing in the institution of binary, narrowly defined gender creates an imperative to reach for social standards of attractiveness. Working to comply with the expectations of dominant culture and attempting to attain privilege by performing these standards or attempting to conform to such standards may provide trans individuals with recognition, inclusion, and protection not otherwise afforded them.

5.1.2.2 Costs of Conformity

Aligning oneself with cisnormative appearance standards has far-reaching impacts for TNB individuals. Visual conformity (also referred to as "passing," or being outwardly perceived as cisgender) is associated with lower risk of physical violence, a reduced risk for experiencing housing insecurity, and fewer periods of being unhoused (Begun & Kattari, 2016). Given the risks TNB people face related to financial instability, being unhoused, and experiences of violence in shelters and transitional living, visual conformity is often simultaneously of heightened importance and more difficult to attain for trans individuals with less class privilege. Malina (2021) has also discussed the ways ever-present threats of physical violence and create an environment in which TNB people take great risks to conform their bodies to appearance standards. Because trans individuals can never fully embody cisnormative appearance standards, attempts to align with the closest possible presentation may be an ongoing goal and struggle throughout life.

TNB individuals who do not or cannot closely conform to these appearance ideals are often simultaneously erased and hyper visible. This phenomenon has been discussed by Black feminists, who explain how Black bodies are pushed out of focus in an attempted erasure while being surveilled and closely scrutinized when they are visible (Johansson, 2021). Of visibility, Johansson (2021) writes, "visibility is a complex force; it can be used as a strategy and tactic of resistance, as well as a mechanism of power" (p. 117). This kind of visibility simultaneously represents both freedom and danger to trans individuals to various degrees depending on intersecting identities that impact social location and proximity to power. Visibility may allow society to see possibilities of trans futures, but those possibilities are narrowly defined and disproportionately impact individuals within TNB communities. Nicolazzo (2019) argues that trans visibility most benefits TNB people who are white, economically secure, and nondisabled while creating a complicated and potentially dangerous awareness of TNB people who face other forms of oppression such as racism, sizeism, classism, and other form of oppression.

Although TNB individuals may make concerted decisions to not attempt conforming to appearance ideals as an act of defiance and challenge to the status quo, trans visibility is also evidence of trans existence and trans joy and has been used as a tool of further oppression by those with social power. On an individual level, trans visibility can be dangerous as long as cisnormative systems are in place that allow and excuse cissexism and violence against TNB individuals. In a social context that rewards conformity through decreased stigma and oppression, occupying a body that cannot fit the standards of acceptable appearance may result in an ongoing fraught relationship with both one's body and food.

5.1.2.3 Coping Strategies

Trans trauma and resilience, then, are central to understanding the ways TNB individuals relate to food and their bodies. Structural and enacted stigma, "mundane" trauma, and oppression are all inherently tied to existing in one's body and the way each individual moves through the world around them. Researchers have documented higher rates of eating disorders and more severe eating disorder symptomology among TNB individuals when compared to cisgender peers (Hallward et al., 2022; Rasmussen et al., 2023). Trauma, discrimination, disconnection, a need for safety through passing, insufficient access to quality care, and coping with these experiences have all been highlighted as important factors related to TNB experiences with eating disorders. Some TNB individuals may also experience gender dysphoria, or distress and discomfort due to incongruence between their sex assigned at birth and gender.

Although gender dysphoria has long been pathologized as a diagnosable "disorder," distress is not an abnormal nor a pathological response to experiencing discrepancy and therefore should not be categorized as a mental illness (Ashley, 2021). The role of gender dysphoria in the way some TNB individuals experience eating disorders and body dissatisfaction must be acknowledged but should also not be understood as the sole driving factor of disordered eating among TNB individuals (Brokjøb & Cornelisse, 2022; Harrop et al., 2023; Malina, 2021). Reducing trans experiences with eating disorders down to only being influenced by dysphoria is inaccurate and causes further harm by obscuring the impacts of social systems and limiting the narrative that dictates where resources and time are devoted (Malina, 2021). As such, there are growing calls to further contextualize eating disorders in the daily experiences of discrimination and trauma faced by TNB individuals. It is widely accepted that eating disorders, for some individuals, may be patterns that have emerged as an attempt to cope with significant stressors and trauma.

Understanding eating disorders and related behaviors as coping mechanisms for trauma is a framework that can be readily expanded to TNB-specific experiences. Participants in qualitative research related to TNB experiences with eating disorders have explicitly cited coping as a common theme related to their understanding of how their eating disorder started (Harrop et al., 2023). Participants in this study named social pressure and discrimination as driving factors behind feelings of bodily dissatisfaction, dysphoria, and disconnection. These experiences, driven by social systems that are hostile to trans existence, result in distress and a growing need to cope with associated feelings.

Clinicians have also highlighted the role of trauma-related coping in trans experiences with eating disorders. Protos (2021) highlighted the importance of identifying and addressing the dynamic relationships between dysphoria, identity-based trauma, and coping in a case study of eating disorder treatment with a trans-masculine adolescent. Just as eating disorder behaviors may be initially experienced as helpful in managing difficult emotions related to trauma more broadly, the same function can be said for coping with identity-based trauma. This association may be even stronger among TNB individuals, however, due to other body-based experiences such as dysphoria, proximity or distance from social appearance standards, and potential perceptions of one's body as the driving force behind experiences of trauma.

5.1.2.4 The Impact of Gender Minority Stress

Indeed, gender minority stress has been broadly linked to eating disorder symptoms among TNB individuals (Cusack et al., 2021). The complex relationships between distal and proximal stressors as related to eating disorder symptoms may be difficult to separate, but researchers have specifically emphasized the link between identity-based oppression and trauma and eating disorder symptomology (Urban et al., 2023; Watson et al., 2017). As discussed above, the "mundane traumas" experienced by many TNB individuals have far-reaching impacts. Daily experiences with oppression and disempowerment challenge the ways TNB people connect with their bodies. Since the world in which we live is experienced while being in one's body, repetitive experiences with lack of safety and harm may cause trans individuals to associate being present in one's body with harm. As such, creating separation between oneself and one's body, as is often seen in individuals with eating disorders, may function as an attempt to create safety in an unsafe environment.

Constant exposure to and socialization in a social context that is cissexist also often results in internalization of cissexist beliefs.[1] When this discrimination and beliefs about the wholeness, validity, or worthiness of trans identities is internalized, TNB individuals often blame themselves for the trauma and discrimination they experience. Cissexism and discrimination also often propose trans identity as the cause of experienced harm. As such, TNB individuals who experience internalization of these beliefs may further distance themselves from their body to protect themselves from more intense feelings related to cissexism. Disconnection from one's body in this sense, then, may lower the threshold for engaging in self-harm and prevent interoception that helps individuals understand what their bodies may need. A decreased ability to connect with and receive signals from one's body due to internalized cissexism and disempowerment also increases the risk for eating disorders among TNB individuals (Malina, 2021).

In light of systems actively working to erase or eliminate trans existence, eating disorder symptoms among TNB individuals unfortunately are not surprising, but they are not the end of the story. Trans joy still exists where TNB individuals are able to create safety. Gender euphoria still works to counteract cissexist, racist norms that dictate the ideal body. However, rising levels of openly hostile discrimination and increasingly restrictive access to gender affirming care threaten safety and access to services that optimize health and reduce mortality of disordered eating in TNB populations. As states, cities, and other jurisdictions work to further degrade the health of TNB people, resilience in the face of immense oppression is likely to become an even more vital pursuit for practitioners, researchers, scholars, and TNB communities.

5.2 Implications

5.2.1 Implications for Understanding Family Resilience

Resilience conceptualized through a third wave lens takes into account behaviors, beliefs, and interpersonal interactions at multiple levels and across multiple systems (Henry et al., 2015). For example, at the individual level TNB people possess individual resilience skills such as hope, self-acceptance, and identity pride (Matsuno & Israel, 2018). At the group level, TNB people may develop and benefit from community belonging, involvement in transgender activism, and the opportunity to be a role model (Matsuno & Israel, 2018). Sometimes resilience at multiple levels

[1] Although this phenomenon is often referred to as "internalized transphobia," we use the term "internalized cissexism" here to explicitly name that cissexist discrimination, not a fear of trans persons (as the term transphobia may imply), is the driving force behind this harm.

enables TNB people to fight systemic oppression directly by adapting in response to discrimination and marginalization. For example, engagement in trans activism and identity as a role model may allow a TNB person to reclaim anti-TNB insults as sources of pride and community identity. At other times, TNB people are forced to call on complex combinations of resilience factors to recover from discrimination and oppression.

Resistance is one of those complex (and so far, understudied) forms of resilience, or steps beyond resilience (Robinson & Schmitz, 2021). When TNB people resist oppression, they move beyond survival and/or coping by reclaiming power for themselves. Resistance involves a refusal to be subjugated, scapegoated, or made responsible for problems (e.g., sexism, racism, heterosexism) that originate in society. For example, resistant TNB people, scholars, treatment providers, and others acknowledge that disordered eating and body image issues are a societal problem. They note that people of all genders suffer from gender-focused oppression and that the illness rests with society, even if emerging research indicates that TNB people are uniquely and disproportionately impacted by dominant beliefs about ideal bodies.

Resistance as a resilience fostering act enables providers, scholars, and TNB people themselves to strike the essential balance between embracing queer beauty, gender euphoria, and trans liberation while also acknowledging that oppression has a very real and powerful impact on TNB people that must be addressed. It expands the work of saving TNB people's lives from a damage-centered, individual-focused task to an effort that encompasses sociocultural contexts, interpersonal relationships, community building, and family-based healing. Emerging research indicates that, for example, family support is one of the most curative factors for TNB youth with disordered eating (Watson et al., 2017).

Breakout Box 5.1: A Parent's Perspective

My daughter's assigned sex at birth was male. As early as 2, we always knew that she was more feminine. The experience of a lot of parents of a trans daughter might think they have a gay son because they have more feminine characteristics. This was my experience. She liked to play dolls and dress up, but we didn't believe that meant much of anything. We weren't conservative in our ideas about gender roles and expression. Around 8 or 9 years old she started saying "I think I am gender neutral." She had read a book with a character who was gender fluid, which I believe to be one of her first encounters with someone identifying in a way that was different than their gender assigned at birth. She had always said things like "I wish I were a girl" or "I should've been a girl" but even as an open-minded parent I didn't understand what that meant. Around 10 or 11 years old, she was often mistaken for a girl because she presented in a very feminine way. I would try to gently correct them because I didn't want her to feel like she was being misgendered. One time at a grocery store the cashier said something like "You little princess" to which I gently responded that my child was a boy. When we left the store, my daughter told me she didn't want me to correct people anymore and that she was okay with people assuming she was a girl. This was one of the first times I understood that she felt more comfortable identifying as a girl. Shortly after this, she sewed herself a dress she could wear and told me that she was wearing it out. She said she wanted to buy her clothes from the girls' section, and she didn't want anyone to think she was a boy ever again. This is when I got it and understood that she was transgender. Initially, I was scared for her. We lived in rural Oklahoma and in my eyes, everyone was going to find out and attack her. She was raised to trust the world but now I feared for her safety. I began googling and mainly found information on Transgender Remembrance Day. The effect the stigmatization has on mental health is so heavy that a disproportionate number of trans people resort to taking their own lives to escape the constant feeling of rejection and unsafety. That terrified me but I don't believe in living in fear, so I tried not to convey that to my daughter. There was one time that she made a shirt that said, "I'm trans and if you are too you're safe with me." I felt obligated as her parent to tell her that people might be rude because they don't understand her shirt. I let her know that I'll be there with her and that I support her, but I just wanted to have the conversation. She told me that she feels really lucky because she gets to be who she is, and she wants to be brave so others can feel safe too. Things got trickier in the teenage years as they do for many. When she first came out, she was comfortable with everyone knowing she was out. As a teenager, she passed as a girl so there was less confusion from others. However, she then had to decide whether or not to come out to people who didn't know her from before. Was she living her truth if they didn't know? Throughout puberty, she had a disconnect from her body due to certain parts not reflecting who she was inside. To feel like she can process who she knows herself to be, she removes herself from her body. She is aware of her body but I do not believe this to be unique to her as a trans girl. This is something girls deal with often, but being trans and having that additional layer of unhappiness with your body makes it much more complicated. Her decision to come out became my responsibility to share because she was so young at the time. She was so brave and fearless, she didn't know anybody like her but she did everything in her power to be her true self. Her bravery changed my life and made me think in different ways. We have been on this path together and one painful thing is that I cannot fix anything for her. As a parent, it still hurts to watch your child suffer or feel scared, even if they are surrounded by the support of their immediate family. Not because being trans is difficult or a challenge per se, but because of how the world treats them. Supporting your child does not mean having all the answers or even understanding, it means listening to your child and making sure they know you are in their corner. It takes great bravery for your child to come out. Listen to what your child has to say and believe it.

—Mother of a transgender daughter

As was established in this chapter, identity-based trauma and micro-oppressions are powerful because of their ability to compound, accumulate, and slowly eat away at the health of TNB people. Disordered eating and body image concerns surface in TNB populations over time and may be the result of the constant impact of cissexist body ideals, oppression-based trauma, a desire to be accepted and seen, and social rejection writ large. However, we would also suggest that the power of resistance and resilience is cumulative, too. Like muscles under the weight of a dumbbell, the more TNB people build their resistance strategies, the more they hold up under the immense weight of discrimination and marginalization aimed at keeping TNB people sick. By leveraging resistance, identifying its benefits, and cultivating its practice in TNB people with disordered eating and body image concerns, we not only cure society's problems as they express themselves in the individual, but we also envision a world in which society itself is changed for the better. As third wave resilience models indicate, societal change is necessary if sustained healing and the mortality rates associated with disordered eating and body image concerns are to be consistently reduced.

5.2.2 Implications for Practice

Understanding the sociocultural context of TNB lives and distress has profound implications for how clinicians engage with those seeking mental healthcare. When TNB individuals present for treatment, practitioners will benefit from seeing members of these communities not as isolated, weakened individuals with disorders but as resilient, powerful, capable individuals beset by laws, policies, social expectations, and interpersonal dynamics aimed at keeping them unwell. This perspective also emphasizes the necessity that treatment experiences do not contribute to oppression-based harm—clinicians and care systems must commit to not worsening the issues they are aiming to help resolve. Practically, this means working hard to avoid misgendering and other signals of non-affirmation and identity invalidation; protecting against cissexism, racism, weight stigma, and other forms of enacted stigma across interaction points in a healthcare system; and ensuring that clients feel a sense of belonging, ideally amplified by having diverse staff that include BIPOC (Black, Indigenous, People of Color) and TNB individuals.

Broadly, because the multiple systems of oppression TNB individuals face is best confronted with the duality of direct acknowledgment of harm and suffering joined with resilience and resistance, clinical practice should also focus on recognizing and validating TNB people's trauma and its impacts, developing and strengthening existing protective factors, building helpful alternative coping capacities, and fostering resistance. That work begins with training and equipping resistant, trauma-informed, affirming practitioners who are prepared to treat TNB people (and clients in general) using a sociocultural, systems-based understanding of the development of disordered eating. Resistance confronts bias and refuses to comply with racism, sexism, cissexism, sizeism, ableism, and other forms of oppression. Clinically, this involves uprooting internalized biases and self-oppressive messages that lie at the core of disordered eating that develops in response to trauma and will likely require that practitioners continuously examine and deconstruct this for themselves as well. Challenging appearance standards, racism, cissexism, heterosexism, ableism, and other forms of oppression is central to working alongside TNB individuals in therapy.

Trauma-informed care with TNB clients is manifold. Being trauma-informed means being able to recognize and name clients' sources and impacts of trauma and harm. Being trauma informed also involves the use of transparent, collaborative, empowering, safety-centered approaches that avoid retraumatization and minimizes the triggering of trauma responses, and may simultaneously facilitate healing of the trauma itself, even while focus may be more specifically on other facets of the presenting concern (e.g., eating behaviors; see Barr et al., in press; Minshew, 2022, for more guidance on incorporating trauma-informed care into work with TNB individuals).

Gender affirming practices during screening and treatment are critical. Concrete examples of gender affirming practices within clinical care may include using TNB-appropriate measures for screening and symptom measurement, using inclusive intake forms, creating and continually updating gender affirming referrals for interdisciplinary care, and more. We underline community members, scholars, and practitioners (recognizing these are not mutually exclusive groups) within the eating disorder field who have specifically called for education and training in these areas and beyond (Goetz & Wolk, 2023; Hartman-Munick et al., 2021; White et al., 2022). Truly gender affirming eating disorder care also means creating spaces that are trauma informed, anti-racist, and weight-inclusive (Goetz & Wolk, 2023; White et al., 2022). As we reviewed, gender dysphoria can be a contributing or exacerbating factor in disordered eating behaviors; efforts to reduce incongruence via social and medical affirmation steps (i.e., gender transition) can be impactful for both a person's overall well-being and their disordered eating specifically. Importantly, while acknowledging this critical component of a treatment plan for trans individuals who wish to pursue medical affirmation, it is important to note that not all TNB individuals desire all or any components of medical affirmation. We also advocate against the damage-focused models which treat gender dysphoria as the core of a TNB person's problem and emphasize the ways in which sociocultural context both separately and through interaction with dysphoria can contribute to distress and disordered eating (Goldbach et al., 2023).

In paying attention to the broader systems affecting the development and maintenance of disordered eating behaviors (White et al., 2022), advocates for health and wellness must recognize the ways that emerging laws also contribute to the psychosocial and physical trauma TNB people endure (e.g., Brightman et al., 2023), enforcing and sustaining the sorts of isolation, shame, and healthcare dysfunction that amplify disordered eating behaviors in TNB populations and other marginalized communities. Anti-trans laws that have been passed reflect growing hostility toward trans individuals and create further legal barriers to safety and acceptance in states where laws have been enacted. Further, TNB people who live in states where anti-trans laws have not been passed may still be impacted by growing anti-trans sentiment.

Clinical work will also benefit from incorporating interventions and approaches directly targeting the further development of resilience in clients. While there are valid critiques of overly focusing on resilience (as opposed to resistance to the contexts that require resilience), we know that resilience can be liberatory when clients' reality is that of ongoing oppression and harm (French et al., 2020). When practitioners abandon damage-focused models of care in favor of person-in-context or sociocultural understandings, they will be better positioned to identify the distress tolerance capacity, coping skills, and resilience potential already present in their clients, can reflect these back and strengthen them, and also help them discover or build other dimensions of resilience. We also know that people who have intersecting identities and/or experience intersecting oppressions often experience stress and trauma and understand recovery and resilience in individually unique ways that are influenced by intersecting experiences (Bryant-Davis, 2019; Jackson et al., 2020). As such, it is important clinicians help clients develop sources of resilience unique to those intersections and individual need. For more guidance on centering resilience in clinical practice, we recommend reading the Trans Resilience Intervention Model (Matsuno & Israel, 2018) and work on the Radical Healing model for BIPOC individuals (French et al., 2020), including radical hope in the face of oppression (Mosley et al., 2020).

Resilience-focused, socioculturally informed approaches to care also make space for gender euphoria and positive emotions, not just as goals or artifacts of successful care, but as preexisting tools that can be utilized or built upon for healing. Socioculturally grounded, effective disordered eating care for TNB people has the potential of not only amplifying gender euphoria, but of recognizing its existence and potential in the treatment process. Focusing on resilience also enables providers and others to get out of the way of TNB people's pursuit of their own care, especially when laws aimed at restricting access are on the rise. When providers trust TNB people, they are less likely to engage in gatekeeping, perpetuate underdiagnosis of disordered eating and other presenting concerns, and/or to reinforce limiting narratives that dismiss or mischaracterize the lives and experiences of TNB people (see Malina, 2021).

Aside from what happens in and around clinical treatment, a sociocultural approach to disordered eating treatment in TNB people includes a call to action and advocacy. Readers are likely to notice that resistance to oppression and challenging toxic societal norms are common themes in this chapter. However, socioculturally informed therapists go beyond simply implying resistance to repressive laws, policies, and societal beliefs. Resilience-focused practitioners, researchers, and scholars are also advocates for TNB people against the systems and norms that increase distress and necessitate coping and survival in the first place (Ashley & Dominguez, 2021). The systems awareness introduced by third wave resilience includes not only treatment and disease management but also prevention. Effective providers are called not only to treat disordered eating after the fact, but also to take action to prevent its development in the first place.

In sum, a systems-focused, resilience-based model of work with the TNB individuals experiencing disordered eating honors the harmful experiences a person has endured while centering their healing potential and organizing other clinically relevant factors around that capacity for resilience. Engaging in this work requires an understanding of the ways oppression and trauma impact TNB individuals and eating disorders, as well as the ways in which TNB individuals and communities resist and are resilient to these experiences. This chapter can serve as a starting point for education, but ongoing, in-depth learning is necessary to provide the best care possible. We encourage practitioners to read some of the more clinically focused texts we have highlighted in this section and pursue training and supervision to continue their education in this area meaningfully.

5.3 Conclusion and Future Directions

Third wave resilience models are key to reducing lethal behaviors and experiences that impact TNB people, such as disordered eating and body image concerns. Comprehensive, multisystem, multilevel models allow for the essential, simultaneous awareness of both oppressive forces and resilience potential in marginalized TNB populations. They also hint at the beginnings of a potential fourth wave that could facilitate not only systems-informed responses to oppression, but systems-driven resistance to oppression that strategically reclaims, reframes, and takes back power and agency for TNB people. Whatever the case, this chapter calls researchers, scholars, practitioners and others to open up more space in the disordered eating and body image literature for gender euphoria, trans liberation, community building, and affirming practices.

Toward that end, researchers are likely to benefit from incorporating the sorts of complexity contained in third wave resilience theories into their research design and practice. For example, the use of Community-Based Participatory Action research methods may open up more space for TNB people's voices in work that is generally conducted about them rather than with them. They may also benefit from shifting away from damage-centered, individual-oriented research design to more intersectional, community-focused investigations of sociocultural context and its role in maladaptive forms of coping. As researchers design measures specific to TNB communities, they may discover new aspects of distress and healing that uniquely contribute to disordered eating and body image that branch outside of current damage-based models. Resilience and resistance measures, scales, and design considerations are likely to bolster and augment future disordered eating and body image studies.

Scholars may benefit from striking a more appropriate balance between writing about/endorsing damage-based models and uplifting resilience and resistance strategies. Activists for gender equity continue to call for a greater acknowledgment in textbooks, syllabi, and other curricula of the strength, beauty, adaptability, and achievements of TNB people (Knutson et al., 2022). Scholars sometimes determine what story will be told about the populations they write, teach, and provide trainings about. We hope that this chapter will shine a light on the critical issues associated with working from damage-based assumptions when discussing TNB people's health and well-being. This awareness may motivate scholars to tell new stories about TNB people, stories that counteract the discrimination and trauma that reinforce disordered eating and body image concerns. The result is likely to be reductions in disordered eating and body image concerns.

Practitioners and community partners who are focused on empowering and uplifting TNB populations are likely well aware of the sorts of compound trauma and discrimination that harry TNB communities. As noted in this chapter, it is important not to lose sight of and/or ignore the very real oppression that TNB people experience. It is also vitally important not to lose sight of and/or ignore the incredible power of trans liberation. Community work and TNB affirming practice can be emotionally taxing, especially in states where laws are being passed to restrict TNB affirming care and other rights for TNB people. Against such oppressive backdrops, it is vitally important for advocates to never lose sight of the power and life-saving nature of their work. Just as the drip, drip of oppression acts as an acid in the lives of TNB people, resistance, resilience, and hope have a powerful compound effect in the battle against disordered eating and body image concerns in TNB communities.

In closing, we acknowledge that liberation implies imprisonment, resilience implies oppression, and resistance evokes images of attack. As we noted earlier in this chapter, many of these experiences go hand in hand. However, we hope to leave you with the awareness that the converse is true. Research on imprisonment is nothing without the possibility of liberation. Oppression calls for the possibility of liberation. Attack demands resistance. As we envision a future in which TNB people suffer at lower rates from disordered eating and body image concerns, we encourage you to join us in work defined by liberation, resilience, and resistance. As demonstrated in the third wave of family resilience, it is no longer sufficient to focus on damage and individual suffering. We are in this together and the responsibility for a better world lies in our work as a community.

Discussion Questions

1. How do the concepts of liberation, resilience, and resistance apply to your area of work or research?
2. In what ways can researchers and practitioners incorporate intersectional approaches into studies of and work with disordered eating and body image among TNB populations? What specific sociocultural factors should be considered?
3. For practitioners working with TNB populations, what strategies can be implemented to foster resilience while addressing the realities of trauma and discrimination?

4. What impact does the language used in research and practice have on the perceptions of TNB individuals? How can language be used to empower rather than perpetuate stigma?
5. How can professionals ensure they are culturally competent when working with TNB individuals? What training or resources might be necessary to enhance their understanding of TNB experiences and challenges.

References

Ashley, F., & Domínguez, S. (2021). Transgender healthcare does not stop at the doorstep of the clinic. *The American Journal of Medicine, 134*(2), 158–160. https://doi.org/10.1016/j.amjmed.2020.09.030

Ashley, F. (2021). The misuse of gender dysphoria: Toward greater conceptual clarity in transgender health. *Perspectives on Psychological Science, 16*(6), 1159–1164. https://doi.org/10.1177/1745691619872987

Barr, S. M. (2018). *Understanding the relationship between anti-transgender bias, non-affirmation, and post-traumatic stress: A model of internalized transphobia-mediated post-traumatic stress* [Doctoral dissertation, University of Louisville] . Electronic Theses and Dissertations. Paper 3106. https://doi.org/10.18297/etd/3106

Barr, S. M., Cory, J., Dockery, G., Sevelius, J., & Torres, D. (in press). Trauma-informed mental health care for transgender and gender diverse communities. In T. Goetz & A. Keuroghlian (Eds.), *Gender-affirming psychiatric care for transgender and gender diverse people*. American Psychiatry Association Press.

Barr, S. M., Snyder, K. E., Adelson, J. L., & Budge, S. L. (2021). Posttraumatic stress in the trans community: The roles of anti-transgender bias, non-affirmation, and internalized transphobia. *Psychology of Sexual Orientation and Gender Diversity, 9*, 410–421. https://doi.org/10.1037/sgd0000500

Begun, S., & Kattari, S. K. (2016). Conforming for survival: Associations between transgender visual conformity/passing and homelessness experiences. *Journal of Gay & Lesbian Social Services, 28*(1), 54–66. https://doi.org/10.1080/10538720.2016.1125821

Bowleg, L., Malekzadeh, A. N., AuBuchon, K., Ghabrial, M., & Bauer, G. R. (2023). Rare exemplars and missed opportunities: Intersectionality within current sexual and gender diversity research and scholarship in psychology. *Current Opinion in Psychology, 49*. https://doi.org/10.1016/j.copsyc.2022.101511

Briere, J., & Spinazzola, J. (2005). Phenomenology and psychological assessment of complex posttraumatic states. *Journal of Traumatic Stress: Official Publication of The International Society for Traumatic Stress Studies, 18*(5), 401–412. https://doi.org/10.1002/jts.20048

Brokjøb, L. G., & Cornelissen, K. K. (2022). Internalizing minority stress: Gender dysphoria, minority stress, and psychopathology in a Norwegian transgender population. *Psychology of Sexual Orientation and Gender Diversity, 9*(3), 272–286. https://doi.org/10.1037/sgd0000480

Brown, L. S. (2008). *Cultural competence in trauma therapy: Beyond the flashback*. American Psychological Association. https://doi.org/10.1037/11752-000

Brightman, S., Lenning, E., Lurie, K. J., & DeJong, C. (2023). Anti-transgender ideology, laws, and homicide: An analysis of the trifecta of violence. *Homicide Studies*, advance online publication. https://doi.org/10.1177/10887679231201803

Bryant-Davis, T. (2019). The cultural context of trauma recovery: Considering the posttraumatic stress disorder practice guideline and intersectionality. *Psychotherapy, 56*(3), 400. https://doi.org/10.1037/pst0000241

Burnes, T. R., Singh, A. A., Harper, A. J., Harper, B., Maxon-Kann, W., Pickering, D. L., Moundas, S., Scofield, T. R., Roan, A., & Hosea, J. (2010). American Counseling Association competencies for counseling with transgender clients. *Journal of LGBT Issues in Counseling, 4*, 135–159. https://doi.org/10.1080/15538605.2010.524839

Chang, S. C., & Singh, A. A. (2016). Affirming psychological practice with transgender and gender nonconforming people of color. *Psychology of Sexual Orientation and Gender Diversity, 3*(2), 140. https://doi.org/10.1037/sgd0000153

Ching, T. H., Lee, S. Y., Chen, J., So, R. P., & Williams, M. T. (2018). A model of intersectional stress and trauma in Asian American sexual and gender minorities. *Psychology of Violence, 8*(6), 657. https://doi.org/10.1037/vio0000204

Colson, A., Shultz, D., & Matsuno, E. (2023). The effects of minority stress and resilience on trauma symptomology among nonbinary adults. In S. Barr (Chair), *Traumatic stress and healing in trans, nonbinary, and gender expansive communities*. (Symposium presented at American Psychological Association Annual Convention, Washington, D.C.).

Cusack, C. E., Cooper, M., Libbey, N., & Galupo, M. P. (2021). Rumination & eating psychopathology among trans and nonbinary individuals: A path analysis integrating minority stress. *Eating Behaviors, 42*, 101544. https://doi.org/10.1016/j.eatbeh.2021.101544

Deliovsky, K. (2008). Normative white femininity: Race, gender, and the politics of beauty. *Atlantis: Critical Studies in Gender, 33*, 49–59. https://atlantisjournal.ca/index.php/atlantis/article/view/429

DuBois, L. Z., & Juster, R. P. (2022). Lived experience and allostatic load among transmasculine people living in the United States. *Psychoneuroendocrinology, 143*, 105849. https://doi.org/10.1016/j.psyneuen.2022.105849

French, B. H., Lewis, J. A., Mosley, D. V., Adames, H. Y., Chavez-Dueñas, N. Y., Chen, G. A., & Neville, H. A. (2020). Toward a psychological framework of radical healing in communities of color. *The Counseling Psychologist, 48*(1), 14–46. https://doi.org/10.1177/0011000019843506

GagnÉ, P., & Tewksbury, R. (1998). Conformity pressures and gender resistance among transgendered individuals. *Social Problems, 45*, 81–101. https://doi.org/10.2307/3097144

Goetz, T. G., & Wolk, C. B. (2023). Moving toward targeted eating disorder care for transgender, non-binary, and gender expansive patients in the United States. *International Journal of Eating Disorders, 56*, 2210–2222. https://doi.org/10.1002/eat.24055

Goldbach, C., Knutson, D., Kler, S., Klooster, D., LeForce, S., & Milton, D. C. (2023). "I owe no one any gender performance": Transgender and nonbinary individuals' experiences of gender dysphoria in bodily, social, and systemic contexts during the Covid-19 Pandemic. *Bulletin of Applied Transgender Studies, 2*(1–2), 27–46. https://doi.org/10.57814/cchg-zz61

Hallward, L., Nagata, J. M., Rodgers, R. F., & Ganson, K. T. (2022). Examination of eating disorder psychopathology across sexual and gender identities among a Canadian sample. *International Journal of Eating Disorders, 56*(3), 604–615. https://doi.org/10.1002/eat.23872

Harrop, E. N., Hecht, H. K., Harner, V., Call, J., & Holloway, B. T. (2023). "How do I exist in this body…that's outside of the norm?" Trans and nonbinary experiences of conformity, coping, and connection in atypical anorexia. *International Journal of Environmental Research and Public Health, 20*(2), 1156. https://doi.org/10.3390/ijerph20021156

Hartman-Munick, S. M., Silverstein, S., Guss, C. G., Lopez, E., Calzo, J. P., & Gordon, A. R. (2021). Eating disorder screening and treatment experiences in transgender and gender diverse young adults. *Eating Behaviors, 42*, 101517. https://doi.org/10.1016/j.eatbeh.2021.101517

Henry, C. S., Sheffield Morris, A., & Harrist, A. W. (2015). Family resilience: Moving into the third wave. *Family Relations, 64*(1), 22–43. https://doi.org/10.1111/fare.12106

Herman, J. L. (1992). Complex PTSD: A syndrome in survivors of prolonged and repeated trauma. *Journal of Traumatic Stress, 5*(3), 377–391. https://doi.org/10.1002/jts.2490050305

Herman, J. L. (2015). *Trauma and recovery: The aftermath of violence – from domestic abuse to political terror* (2nd ed.). Basic Books.

Jackson, S. D., Mohr, J. J., Sarno, E. L., Kindahl, A. M., & Jones, I. L. (2020). Intersectional experiences, stigma-related stress, and psychological health among Black LGBQ individuals. *Journal of Consulting and Clinical Psychology, 88*(5), 416. https://doi.org/10.1037/ccp0000489

Johansson, A. (2021). Fat, black and unapologetic: Body positive activism beyond white, neoliberal rights discourses. In E. Alm, L. Berg, M. Lundahl Hero, P. Laskar, L. Martinsson, D. Mulinari, & C. Wasshede (Eds.), *Pluralistic struggles in gender, sexuality and coloniality: Challenging Swedish exceptionalism.* Springer International. https://doi.org/10.1007/978-3-030-47432-4

Knutson, D., Matsuno, E., Goldbach, C., Hashtpari, H., & Smith, N. G. (2022). Advocating for transgender and nonbinary affirmative spaces in graduate education. *Higher Education, 83*(2), 461–479. https://doi.org/10.1007/s10734-020-00673-5

Levitt, H. M., Kehoe, K. A., & Hand, A. B. (2023). Beyond minority stress: Toward a multidimensional psychology of trans/nonbinary gender. *Current Opinion in Psychology, 49*, 101515. https://doi.org/10.1016/j.copsyc.2022.101515

Malatino, H. (2022). *Side affects: On being trans and feeling bad.* U of Minnesota Press.

Malina, S. (2021). Unique causes and manifestations of eating disorders within transgender populations. *Columbia Social Work Review, 19*(1), 138–157. https://doi.org/10.52214/cswr.v19i1.7241

Maroney, M. R., & Horne, S. G. (2022). "Tuned into a different channel": Autistic transgender adults' experiences of intersectional stigma. *Journal of Counseling Psychology, 69*(6), 761. https://doi.org/10.1037/cou0000639

Matsuno, E., & Israel, T. (2018). Psychological interventions promoting resilience among transgender individuals; Transgender Resilience Intervention Model (TRIM). *The Counseling Psychologist, 46*(5), 632–655. https://doi.org/10.1177/0011000018787261

Minshew, R. (2022). *Treating trauma in trans people: An intersectional, phase-based approach.* Taylor & Francis. https://doi.org/10.4324/9781003140740

Mosley, D. V., Neville, H. A., Chavez-Dueñas, N. Y., Adames, H. Y., Lewis, J. A., & French, B. H. (2020). Radical hope in revolting times: Proposing a culturally relevant psychological framework. *Social and Personality Psychology Compass, 14*(1), e12512. https://doi.org/10.1111/spc3.12512

Nicolazzo, Z. (2019). Visibility alone will not save us: Leveraging invisibility as a possibility for liberatory pedagogical practice. In *Queer, trans, and intersectional theory in educational practice* (pp. 120–132). Routledge.

Protos, K. (2021). Restricting the gendered body: Understanding the trans-masculine adolescent with anorexia. *Clinical Social Work Journal, 49*(3), 380–390. https://doi.org/10.1007/s10615-020-00758-9

Puckett, J. A. (2019). An ecological approach to therapy with gender minorities. *Cognitive and Behavioral Practice, 26*(4), 647–655. https://doi.org/10.1016/j.cbpra.2019.08.002

Puckett, J. A., Price, S. F., Mocarski, R., Mustanski, B., & Newcomb, M. E. (2022). Transgender and gender diverse individuals' daily experiences of rumination. *American Journal of Orthopsychiatry, 92*(5), 540. https://doi.org/10.1037/ort0000636

Rasmussen, S. M., Dalgaard, M. K., Roloff, M., Pinholt, M., Skrubbeltrang, C., Clausen, L., & Kjaersdam Telléus, G. (2023). Eating disorder symptomatology among transgender individuals: A systematic review and meta-analysis. *Journal of Eating Disorders, 11*(1), 84. https://doi.org/10.1186/s40337-023-00806-y

Reisner, S. L., White Hughto, J. M., Gamarel, K. E., Keuroghlian, A. S., Mizock, L., & Pachankis, J. E. (2016). Discriminatory experiences associated with Posttraumatic Stress Disorder symptoms among transgender adults. *Journal of Counseling Psychology, 63*(5), 1–12. https://doi.org/10.1037/cou0000143

Richmond, K. A., Burnes, T., & Carroll, K. (2012). Lost in translation: Interpreting systems of trauma for transgender clients. *Traumatology, 18*(1), 45–57. https://doi.org/10.1177/1534765610396726

Richmond, K., Burnes, T. R., Singh, A. A., & Ferrara, M. (2017). Assessment and treatment of trauma with TGNC clients: A feminist approach. In D. L. McGuire & J. M. Anderson (Eds.),

Affirmative counseling and psychological practice with transgender and gender nonconforming clients (pp. 191–212). American Psychological Association. https://doi.org/10.1037/14957-010

Robinson, B. A., & Schmitz, R. M. (2021). Beyond resilience: Resistance in the lives of LGBTQ+ youth. *Sociology. Compass, 15*(12). https://doi.org/10.1111/soc4.12947

Root, M. P. (1992). Reconstructing the impact of trauma on personality. In L. S. Brown & M. Ballou (Eds.), *Personality and psychopathology: Feminist reappraisals* (pp. 229–265). Guilford Press.

Tan, K. K., Treharne, G. J., Ellis, S. J., Schmidt, J. M., & Veale, J. F. (2019). Gender minority stress: A critical review. *Journal of Homosexuality, 67*, 1471–1489. https://doi.org/10.1080/00918369.2019.1591789

Urban, B., Knutson, D., Klooster, D., & Soper, J. (2023). Social and contextual influences on eating pathology in transgender and nonbinary adults. *Eating Disorders, 31*(4), 301–319. https://doi.org/10.1080/10640266.2022.2135715

Watson, R. J., Veale, J. F., & Saewyc, E. M. (2017). Disordered eating behaviors among transgender youth: Probability profiles from risk and protective factors. *International Journal of Eating Disorders, 50*, 515–522. https://doi.org/10.1002/eat.22627

Wesp, L. M., Malcoe, L. H., Elliott, A., & Poteat, T. (2019). Intersectionality research for transgender health justice: A theory-driven conceptual framework for structural analysis of transgender health inequities. *Transgender Health, 4*(1), 287–296. https://doi.org/10.1089/trgh.2019.0039

Wesson, P., Vittinghoff, E., Turner, C., Arayasirikul, S., McFarland, W., & Wilson, E. (2021). Intercategorical and intracategorical experiences of discrimination and HIV prevalence among transgender women in San Francisco, CA: A quantitative intersectionality analysis. *American Journal of Public Health, 111*(3), 446–456. https://doi.org/10.2105/AJPH.2020.306055

White, M., Jones, S., & Joy, P. (2022). Safe, seen, and supported: Navigating eating disorders recovery in the 2SLGBTQ+ communities. *Canadian Journal of Dietetic Practice and Research, 84*, 84–92. https://doi.org/10.3148/cjdpr-2022-033

Zimman, L. (2019). Trans self-identification and the language of neoliberal selfhood: Agency, power, and the limits of monologic discourse. *International Journal of the Sociology of Language, 256*, 147–175. https://doi.org/10.1515/ijsl-2018-2016

Chapter 6
Can Food Environments Make or Break Your Healthy Eating Habits?

Jillian M. Joyce, Pamela Gonzalez Sanchez, and Kristen McClanahan

According to nationally representative data for US adults and children, our diets are in need of significant improvement (U.S. Department of Agriculture, Food and Nutrition Service, Center for Nutrition Policy and Promotion, 2023). Data indicate that children aged 2–18 years have a dietary quality score of 54/100, adults aged 19–59 have a score of 57/100, and adults aged 60 years and older have a score of 61/100. Scores below 50 indicate poor dietary quality, 50–79 indicate need for improvement, and 80–100 indicate good dietary quality (Gibson, 2005). Considering these scores fall between 50 and 79 and some are close to 50, US dietary quality is quite low and improvement is needed.

Improving dietary quality scores is incredibly important, as it has academic implications for children and health implications for the whole family. High dietary quality among children is associated with lower risk of obesity, numerous chronic diseases, and mortality from chronic disease as an adult (Perry et al., 2015), predicts their dietary quality as an adult (Marshall et al., 2014), and is associated with reduced absenteeism and improved on-task time, alertness, science and English class performance, and overall grade point average (Haapala et al., 2015). High dietary quality among adults is associated with reduced obesity, cardiovascular disease, type 2 diabetes, and numerous types of cancer (Alkerwi, 2014; Asghari et al., 2017). Dietary quality is also consistently and positively associated with measures of mental health (Collins et al., 2020; Jacka et al., 2011; Opie et al., 2015).

Dietary quality scores in the United States are in need of improvement and have been for decades, remaining mostly unchanged, despite individual, community, and national level interventions. Thus, the need exists for novel strategies that look

J. M. Joyce (✉) · P. G. Sanchez · K. McClanahan
Department of Nutritional Sciences, Oklahoma State University, Stillwater, OK, USA

Tactical Fitness and Nutrition Lab, Oklahoma State University, Stillwater, OK, USA
e-mail: jill.joyce@okstate.edu

G. Welch et al. (eds.), *Stress, Resilience, and Healthy Relationships with Food and Family*, Emerging Issues in Family and Individual Resilience,
https://doi.org/10.1007/978-3-031-98937-7_6

beyond the current focus of existing interventions. Food environments are one such area of novel and increasing focus. Current food environments are designed to overwhelm our willpower and drive us toward less healthy food choices (DellaVigna, 2009; Thaler & Sunstein, 2009). However, public health nutrition practitioners are learning to redesign the environment in which we make daily food choices to make healthier choices easier (Thaler & Sunstein, 2009). This redesign is done through choice architecture, which employs behavioral economics or nudge strategies.

With a national need to improve nutrition habits of Americans, as well as a need for novel approaches to make eating healthier easier, this critical review of the literature related to food environments and choice architecture aims to (a) define various food environments in which we live and make food decisions as families, (b) define choice architecture, and (c) describe how to use behavioral economics or nudge strategies to improve dietary quality of family eating patterns.

6.1 Dietary Quality: Definition and Importance

Dietary quality assesses how healthy a dietary pattern is based on how closely that pattern aligns with scientific or government recommendations for a healthy diet (Wirt & Collins, 2009). One of the most commonly used, valid, and reliable tools for assessing dietary quality is the Healthy Eating Index (HEI), which uses the Dietary Guidelines for Americans (DGA) as the recommendation with which to compare dietary patterns for alignment. A higher HEI score indicates better alignment with the DGA and thus higher dietary quality (Shams-White et al., 2023; Wirt & Collins, 2009). As mentioned above, we can further categorize HEI scores for dietary quality into three categories—below 50 indicates poor dietary quality, 50–79 indicates need for improvement, and 80–100 indicates good dietary quality (Gibson, 2005).

Dietary quality assessment has gained increasing attention in the literature and public health nutrition practice, due to the ever-increasing prevalence of childhood overweight and obesity, the connection between nutrition and obesity, and the need to assess children's dietary quality (Kourlaba & Panagiotakos, 2009; Marshall et al., 2014; Perry et al., 2015; Roman-Vinas et al., 2009). Further adding to this concern is the fact that developing obesity during childhood increases the risk of becoming an adult with obesity (Perry et al., 2015).

Dietary quality is a versatile concept with a wide range of applications across diverse populations making it an ideal focus for health promotion and obesity prevention. For instance, it has been used to predict childhood obesity and to explain the relationship between diet and various health conditions (Kourlaba & Panagiotakos, 2009; Marshall et al., 2014; Perry et al., 2015; Roman-Vinas et al., 2009). Similarly, among the adult population, it has been used to quantify the risk of chronic conditions like certain cancers and cardiovascular disease (Kimokoti & Millen, 2011; Marshall et al., 2014; Perry et al., 2015; Wirth & Collins, 2009).

Moreover, dietary quality provides crucial insights into the connection between parent and child dietary habits. Research has revealed a positive association between parental dietary quality, especially maternal dietary quality, and the dietary quality of children (Beydoun & Wang, 2009; Cheng et al., 2010; Darapheak et al., 2013; Laster et al., 2013; Manios et al., 2009; Marshall et al., 2014; Rauber et al., 2013; Vitolo et al., 2010). Furthermore, poor dietary quality has been associated with factors such as the earlier onset of puberty, a known risk factor for hormone-related cancers, mortality, and insulin resistance. Its impact extends to positive associations with child growth measures as well, particularly in developing nations where the risk of undernutrition remains a significant concern (Cheng et al., 2010; Marshall et al., 2014).

Additionally, studying children's dietary patterns holds significant public health implications, as the results are often more easily translated into public health messages than research focused on specific foods or nutrients. This information can also serve essential epidemiological purposes (Haapala et al., 2015; Perry et al., 2015). Thus, the relevance of dietary quality is evident after recognizing some of its diverse approaches among different fields and populations.

Adequate and proper nutrition is not only important for normal physical development in children, but also for normal cognitive development (Florence et al., 2008; Roberts et al., 2022; Haapala et al., 2015; Marshall et al., 2014). There are two main factors, limited food access to nutritious foods and undernutrition, which have been linked to decreased cognitive functions in children and strongly related to poor dietary quality (Arimond & Ruel, 2004; Marshall et al., 2014; Ruel, 2003). Thus, poor diet quality is associated with worse cognitive performance in children. Additionally, this relationship is not limited to children, as dietary quality indices are directly associated with cognition in older adults as well (Haapala et al., 2015).

More specifically, evidence suggests that a poorer adherence to the Mediterranean-style diet leads to poorer academic achievement in children. Low fruit, vegetable, dietary fiber, fish, and cheese intake have also been associated with a lower intelligence quotient, poorer memory, and worse cognitive control in later years. Moreover, a higher consumption of red and processed meats may harm children's cognition. Conversely, a diet rich in fruits (especially berries), vegetables, fish, and high-fiber grain products supports the normal development of children's cognition (Haapala et al., 2015).

In summary, it is evident that dietary quality plays a crucial role in children's physical and cognitive development, and these findings highlight the importance of monitoring dietary quality and promoting healthier eating habits not only in children but also in adults.

6.2 Food Environments

There are countless influences on all health behaviors, and nutrition is no exception. One of those factors, that is often overlooked by patients and practitioners alike, is the environment. The environment broadly impacts many aspects of our health, but especially our health behaviors, through physical design or built environment, social-cultural roles, and socioeconomic status (Lake & Townshend, 2006). As this chapter focuses on food environments, we will narrow our discussion to built environment, under which food environments fall. Elements of the food environment that impact our eating behaviors, and thus nutrition, include food availability, food accessibility, and advertising and marketing, which includes policy and promotion (Centers for Disease Control and Prevention, 2014; Lake & Townshend, 2006).

Two common concepts that highlight the impact of access and availability in macro-level (or community) food environments are food deserts and food swamps (Cooksey-Stowers et al., 2017; Dutko et al., 2012). Food deserts are environments in which there is a lack of access to a variety of healthy, affordable foods (Dutko et al., 2012). Food swamps are environments in which there is excessive access to energy-dense, nutrient-poor foods, especially relative to healthier options (Cooksey-Stowers et al., 2017). Living in food deserts and food swamps both individually are predictors of poor dietary quality, obesity, and negative health outcomes (Cooksey-Stowers et al., 2017; Dutko et al., 2012). Thus, the community food environment you live in greatly impacts your eating habits and thus nutrition and related health outcomes. The next section will describe how micro-level (i.e., inside individual stores and restaurants, home, the office, etc.) food environments impact eating habits.

6.3 Choice Architecture

Choice architecture is defined as the design of an environment in which a choice is made. Where choice architecture connects to health behaviors, especially eating habits, is through nudges. Nudges are changes to the choice architecture in order to influence decision making in a certain way. These concepts may also be collectively referred to as behavioral economics. Currently, food environments are designed to quickly overwhelm willpower surrounding healthy eating. However, there is good news. Choice architecture is a way to encourage change when change is hard. We can redesign the food environment to make the healthy choice the easy choice (Ammerman et al., 2017; DellaVigna, 2009; Thaler & Sunstein, 2009).

How do nudge strategies or behavioral economics work? When we make decisions, we rely on two systems: (1) values and logic systems and (2) automatic and irrational systems (Just & Payne, 2009; Marteau et al., 2011). Unfortunately, the first system, which traditional education targets, requires cognitive capacity to work. As people and families become busier and busier with more on their plates, they use up their limited cognitive capacity by the end of the day, if not sooner (Just & Payne, 2009; Marteau et al., 2011; Payne et al., 2014; Wilson et al., 2016). Thus, we often turn to our automatic, irrational system to make decisions, as this system requires very little cognitive capacity. This automatic system is susceptible to and easily influenced by the environment (Gittelsohn & Lee, 2013; Just & Payne, 2009; Marteau et al., 2011). With this in mind, we should not assume that people make poor food decisions due to lack of willpower, as this is often not the case. Instead, we should realize that food decisions are typically automatic and irrational, especially in times of high stress, going for the easiest choice with the least amount of mental effort needed (Ammerman et al., 2017; Arno & Thomas, 2016; Ensaff et al., 2015; Gittelsohn & Lee, 2013; Just & Payne, 2009; Kraak et al., 2017; Thorndike et al., 2012; van Kleef et al., 2012; Wilson et al., 2016). Public health researchers like Thaler and Sunstein (2009), as well as Just and Payne (2009), realized that if restaurants and stores can capitalize on overwhelming our willpower to drive us toward less healthy food options, then they could turn the tables and rearrange the environment through nudges to drive us toward healthier food options.

There are many nudge strategies that can be used, but to simplify them for use in micro-level environments that patients control (i.e., home and the office), practitioners should focus on three concepts—normal, attractive, and convenient (Ammerman et al., 2017; DellaVigna, 2009; Just and Payne, 2009; Thaler & Sunstein, 2009). Due to the automatic system mentioned earlier, people will eat whatever is normal, attractive, and convenient. Thus, we have six opportunities to nudge individuals toward a healthier diet, which can be found in Table 6.1. With each nudge, we increase the likelihood of an individual eating a healthier diet.

6.4 Implications

6.4.1 Implications for Understanding Family Resilience

As mentioned, people and families are becoming busier and busier with more on their plates. Because of this, they use up their cognitive capacity and turn to their automatic, irrational system to make food decisions for themselves and their families. This automatic system is susceptible to and easily influenced by the environment, which can either make or break our healthy eating plans depending on how that environment is set up. Sticking to a high dietary quality eating pattern results in lower chronic disease risk for all family members, better academic performance for children, and all together a more resilient family. Thus, it is important to find ways to make the healthy choice the easy choice for families. In order to reduce cognitive burden surrounding healthy food decisions for their families, we can encourage families to use behavioral economic strategies and nudge their family members toward healthy eating habits by making healthier food more normal, attractive, and

Table 6.1 Behavioral economic strategies to encourage healthier food consumption

Behavioral economic strategy	Examples
For healthier food items	
More normal	Consistently swap out refined bread for whole grain bread on the grocery list each week Buy bananas each week
More attractive	Place the whole grain bread at eye level in the pantry to catch your eye Display the bananas in an attractive bowl visibly on the countertop
More convenient	Buy pre-sliced bread and make sure it is in the front of the pantry for quick, easy use Place the grab-and-go bananas on a countertop where people regularly pass
For less healthy food items	
Less normal	Only buy cookies on occasion when you really want them Don't keep chips in the house but enjoy them when out from time to time for lunch
Less attractive	Remove the cookies from the bright and colorful package and place them in a non-see-through container Place the chips behind healthier items in the pantry
Less convenient	Put the cookie jar on the top shelf in a kitchen cupboard Put the chips in the back of the pantry behind a closed door

convenient and less healthy food less normal, attractive, and convenient in the places where they spend the majority of their time (e.g., home, work, school).

6.4.2 Implications for Practice and/or Policy

This chapter highlights the importance of considering the environment when families are struggling to implement and stick to healthier habits, especially in busy or stressful situations. Practitioners are advised to ask questions about how the home, work, or school environments may be encouraging continuation of unhealthy habits, and then work with the family to consider how they could rearrange the environments to make healthier habits easier to perform and maintain. It should be noted that this chapter focused on food environment, but these techniques can be applied to an environment surrounding any healthy habit (e.g., cell phone use, physical activity, and smoking).

There are also implications for policy, especially in settings in which individuals have less control. Advocating for wellness policies at work and school can also encourage changes in environments on a larger scale to reach more people. Some examples of potential policies across various environments beyond the home include:

- Keeping countertops free of less healthy foods at a fire station
- Having a fruit bowl instead of a candy dish at the front desk

- Putting unflavored milk in front of chocolate milk in the school cafeteria cooler
- Encouraging activities for celebrations instead of food items in classrooms
- Requiring that half of the options in the vending machines meet healthy nutrition standards

6.5 Conclusion and Future Directions

In conclusion, practitioners need to ensure they consider environments when discussing barriers to change and in helping families make and maintain healthy changes. When new healthy habits are more normal, attractive, and convenient, they become easier choices to make. Most of the research on behavioral economics in public health to this point has been conducted in schools. Despite the concepts translating easily to other environments, more research is needed in home and work environments to confirm their effectiveness. Additionally, most research has been conducted to improve eating patterns and physical activity levels. More research is needed on effectiveness of behavioral economics in implementing and maintaining other healthy lifestyle habits.

Discussion Questions

1. What is the importance of good nutrition to families, and why does it need improvement?
2. What food environments do you live in daily, and how do they influence your dietary quality?
3. How can you use behavioral economics in your daily food environments to improve your dietary quality?
4. How will the information provided today change how you consider nutrition and environments in your professional practice?

References

Alkerwi, A. (2014). Diet quality concept. *Nutrition, 30*, 613–618. https://doi.org/10.1016/j.nut/2013.10.001

Ammerman, A. S., Hartman, T., & DeMarco, M. M. (2017). Behavioral economics and the Supplemental Nutrition Assistance Program: Making the healthy choice the easy choice. *American Journal of Preventive Medicine, 52*(2S2), S145–S150. https://doi.org/10.1016/j.amepre.2016.08.017

Arimond, M., & Ruel, M. T. (2004). Dietary diversity is associated with child nutritional status: Evidence from 11 demographic and Health Surveys. *The Journal of Nutrition, 134*(10), 2579–2585. https://doi.org/10.1093/jn/134.10.2579

Arno, A., & Thomas, S. (2016). The efficacy of nudge theory strategies in influencing adult dietary behaviour: A systematic review and meta-analysis. *BMC Public Health, 16*(1), 676–687. https://doi.org/10.1186/s12889-016-3272-x

Asghari, G., Mirmiran, P., Yuzbashian, E., & Azizi, F. (2017). A systematic review of diet quality indices in relation to obesity. *British Journal of Nutrition, 117*, 1055–1065. https://doi.org/10.1017/s0007114517000915

Beydoun, M. A., & Wang, Y. (2009). Parent–child dietary intake resemblance in the United States: Evidence from a large representative survey. *Social Science & Medicine, 68*(12), 2137–2144. https://doi.org/10.1016/j.socscimed.2009.03.029

Centers for Disease Control and Prevention. (2014, March 6). *General food environment resources*. CDC. https://www.cdc.gov/healthyplaces/healthtopics/healthyfood/general.htm

Cheng, G., Gerlach, S., Libuda, L., Kranz, S., Günther, A. L. B., Karaolis-Danckert, N., Kroke, A., & Buyken, A. E. (2010). Diet quality in childhood is prospectively associated with the timing of puberty but not with body composition at puberty onset. *The Journal of Nutrition, 140*(1), 95–102. https://doi.org/10.3945/jn.109.113365

Collins, S., Dash, S., Allender, S., Jacka, F., & Hoare, E. (2020). Diet and mental health during emerging adulthood: A systematic review. *Emerging Adulthood, 10*(3), 645–659. https://doi.org/10.1177/2167696820943028

Cooksey-Stowers, K., Schwartz, M. B., & Brownell, K. D. (2017). Food swamps predict obesity rates better than food deserts in the United States. *International Journal of Environmental Research and Public Health, 14*(11), 1366–1386. https://doi.org/10.3390/ijerph14111366

Darapheak, C., Takano, T., Kizuki, M., Nakamura, K., & Seino, K. (2013). Consumption of animal source foods and dietary diversity reduce stunting in children in Cambodia. *International Archives of Medicine, 6*(1), 29–40. https://doi.org/10.1186/1755-7682-6-29

DellaVigna, S. (2009). Psychology and economics: Evidence from the field. *Journal of Economic Literature, 47*(2), 315–372. https://doi.org/10.1257/jel.47.2.315

Dutko, P., Ver Ploeg, M., & Farrigan, T. (2012). *Characteristics and influential factors of food deserts (ERR-140)*. U.S. Department of Agriculture, Economic Research Service.

Ensaff, H., Homer, M., Sahota, P., Braybrook, D., Coan, S., & McLeod, H. (2015). Food choice architecture: An intervention in a secondary school and its impact on students' plant-based food choices. *Nutrients, 7*(6), 4426–4437. https://doi.org/10.3390/nu7064426

Florence, M. D., Asbridge, M., & Veugelers, P. J. (2008). Diet quality and academic performance. *Journal of School Health, 78*(4), 209–215. https://doi.org/10.1111/j.1746-1561.2008.00288.x

Gibson, R. S. (2005). *Principles of nutritional assessment* (2nd ed.). Oxford University Press.

Gittelsohn, J., & Lee, K. (2013). Integrating educational, environmental, and behavioral economic strategies may improve the effectiveness of obesity interventions. *Applied Economic Perspectives and Policy, 35*(1), 52–68. https://doi.org/10.1093/aepp/pps044

Haapala, E., Eloranta, A., Venäläinen, T., Schwab, U., Lindi, V., & Lakka, T. (2015). Associations of diet quality with cognition in children – The Physical Activity and Nutrition in Children Study. *British Journal of Nutrition, 114*(7), 1080–1087. https://doi.org/10.1017/s0007114515001634

Jacka, F. N., Mykletun, A., Berk, M., Bjelland, I., & Tell, G. S. (2011). The association between habitual diet quality and the common mental disorders in community-dwelling adults: The Hordaland Health Study. *Psychosomatic Medicine, 73*(6), 483–490. https://doi.org/10.1097/PSY.0b013e318222831a

Just, D. R., & Payne, C. R. (2009). Obesity: Can behavioral economics help? *Annals of Behavioral Medicine, 38*(Suppl 1), S47–S55. https://doi.org/10.1007/s12160-009-9119-2

Kimokoti, R. W., & Millen, B. E. (2011). Diet, the global obesity epidemic, and prevention. *Journal of the American Dietetic Association, 111*(8), 1137–1140. https://doi.org/10.1016/j.jada.2011.05.016

Kourlaba, G., & Panagiotakos, D. B. (2009). Dietary quality indices and human health: A review. *Maturitas, 62*(1), 1–8. https://doi.org/10.1016/j.maturitas.2008.11.021

Kraak, V. I., Englund, T., Misyak, S., & Serrano, E. L. (2017). A novel marketing mix and choice architecture framework to nudge restaurant customers toward healthy food environments to reduce obesity in the United States: A marketing and nudge framework for restaurants. *Obesity Reviews, 18*(8), 852–868. https://doi.org/10.1111/obr.12553

Lake, A., & Townshend, T. (2006). Obesogenic environments: Exploring the built and food environments. *Journal of the Royal Society for the Promotion of Health, 126*(6), 262–267. https://doi.org/10.1177/1466424006070487

Laster, L. E., Lovelady, C. A., West, D. G., Wiltheiss, G. A., Brouwer, R. J. N., Stroo, M., & Østbye, T. (2013). Diet quality of overweight and obese mothers and their preschool children. *Journal of the Academy of Nutrition and Dietetics, 113*(11), 1476–1483. https://doi.org/10.1016/j.jand.2013.05.018

Manios, Y., Kourlaba, G., Kondaki, K., Grammatikaki, E., Birbilis, M., Oikonomou, E., & Roma-Giannikou, E. (2009). Diet quality of preschoolers in Greece based on the healthy eating index: The genesis study. *Journal of the American Dietetic Association, 109*(4), 616–623. https://doi.org/10.1016/j.jada.2008.12.011

Marshall, S., Burrows, T., & Collins, C. E. (2014). Systematic review of diet quality indices and their associations with health-related outcomes in children and adolescents. *Journal of Human Nutrition and Dietetics, 27*(6), 577–598. https://doi.org/10.1111/jhn.12208

Marteau, T. M., Ogilvie, D., Roland, M., Suhrcke, M., & Kelly, M. P. (2011). Judging nudging: Can nudging improve population health? *BMJ, 342*(3), d228–d228. https://doi.org/10.1136/bmj.d228

Opie, R. S., O'Neil, A., Itsiopoulos, C., & Jacka, F. N. (2015). The impact of whole-of-diet interventions on depression and anxiety: A systematic review of randomised controlled trials. *Public Health Nutrition, 18*(11), 2074–2093. https://doi.org/10.1017/S1368980014002614

Payne, C. R., Niculescu, M., Just, D. R., & Kelly, M. P. (2014). Shopper marketing nutrition interventions. *Physiology and Behavior, 136*, 111–120. https://doi.org/10.1016/j.physbeh.2014.03.029

Perry, C., Keane, E., Layte, R., Fitzgerald, A., Perry, I., & Harrington, J. (2015). The use of a dietary quality score as a predictor of childhood overweight and obesity. *BMC Public Health, 15*, 581–590. https://doi.org/10.1186/s12889-015-1907-

Rauber, F., Hoffman, D. J., & Vitolo, M. R. (2013). Diet quality from pre-school to school age in Brazilian children: A 4-year follow-up in a randomised control study. *British Journal of Nutrition, 111*(3), 499–505. https://doi.org/10.1017/s0007114513002857

Roberts, M., Tolar-Peteron, T., Reynolds, A., Wall, C., Reeder, N., Rico Mendez G. (2022). The effects of nutritional interventions on the cognitive development of preschool-age children: A systematic review. *Nutrients, 14*(3), 532. https://doi.org/10.3390/nu1403053210.3390/nu14030532

Roman-Vinas, B., Ribas Barba, L., Ngo, J., Ángel Martínez-González, M., Wijnhoven, T. M., & Serra-Majem, L. (2009). Validity of dietary patterns to assess nutrient intake adequacy. *British Journal of Nutrition, 101*(S2). https://doi.org/10.1017/s0007114509990547

Ruel, M. T. (2003). Operationalizing dietary diversity: A review of measurement issues and research priorities. *The Journal of Nutrition, 133*(11). https://doi.org/10.1093/jn/133.11.3911s

Shams-White, M. M., Pannucci, T. E., Lerman, J., et al. (2023). Healthy Eating Index-2020. Review and update process to reflect the Dietary Guidelines for Americans, 2020-2025. *Journal of the Academy of Nutrition and Dietetics, 123*(9), 1280–1288. https://doi.org/10.1016/j.jand.2023.05.015

Thaler, R., & Sunstein, C. (2009). *Nudge: Improving decisions about health, wealth, and happiness*. Penguin Books.

Thorndike, A. N., Sonnenberg, L., Riis, J., Barraclough, S., & Levy, D. E. (2012). A 2-phase labeling and choice architecture intervention to improve healthy food and beverage choices. *American Journal of Public Health, 102*(3), 527–533. https://doi.org/10.2105/AJPH.2011.300391

U.S. Department of Agriculture, Food and Nutrition Service, Center for Nutrition Policy and Promotion. (2023). *Average Healthy Eating Index-2020 Scores for the U.S. population – total ages 2 and older and by age groups, WWEIA, NHANES 2017-2018.* fns-prod.azureedge.us van Kleef, E., Otten, K., & van Trijp, H. C. (2012). Healthy snacks at the checkout counter: A lab and field study on the impact of shelf arrangement and assortment structure on consumer choices. *BMC Public Health, 12*(1), 1072. https://doi.org/10.1186/1471-2458-12-1072

Vitolo, M. R., Rauber, F., Campagnolo, P. D., Feldens, C. A., & Hoffman, D. J. (2010). Maternal dietary counseling in the first year of life is associated with a higher healthy eating index in childhood. *The Journal of Nutrition, 140*(11), 2002–2007. https://doi.org/10.3945/jn.110.125211

Wilson, A. L., Buckley, E., Buckley, J. D., & Bogomolova, S. (2016). Nudging healthier food and beverage choices through salience and priming. Evidence from a systematic review. *Food Quality and Preference, 51*, 47–64. https://doi.org/10.1016/j.foodqual.2016.02.009

Wirt, A., & Collins, C. E. (2009). Diet quality – what is it and does it matter? *Public Health Nutrition, 12*(12), 2473–2492. https://doi.org/10.1017/s136898000900531x

Index

G. Welch et al. (eds.), *Stress, Resilience, and Healthy Relationships with Food and Family*, Emerging Issues in Family and Individual Resilience,
https://doi.org/10.1007/978-3-031-98937-7

FSC www.fsc.org
MIX
Papier aus verantwortungsvollen Quellen
Paper from responsible sources
FSC® C105338

If you have any concerns about our products,
you can contact us on
ProductSafety@springernature.com

In case Publisher is established outside the EU,
the EU authorized representative is:
Springer Nature Customer Service Center GmbH
Europaplatz 3, 69115 Heidelberg, Germany

Printed by Libri Plureos GmbH
in Hamburg, Germany